THE FOOD CURE

Clinically Proven Antioxidant Foods to Prevent
and Treat Chronic Diseases and Conditions

THE FOOD CURE

Clinically Proven Antioxidant Foods to Prevent and Treat Chronic Diseases and Conditions

MONTE LAI, PH.D.

Former Professor of Biophysics, Medical College of Wisconsin, USA

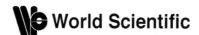 World Scientific

NEW JERSEY · LONDON · SINGAPORE · BEIJING · SHANGHAI · HONG KONG · TAIPEI · CHENNAI · TOKYO

Published by

World Scientific Publishing Co. Pte. Ltd.
5 Toh Tuck Link, Singapore 596224
USA office: 27 Warren Street, Suite 401-402, Hackensack, NJ 07601
UK office: 57 Shelton Street, Covent Garden, London WC2H 9HE

Library of Congress Cataloging-in-Publication Data
Names: Lai, Monte, author.
Title: The food cure : clinically proven antioxidant foods to prevent and
    treat chronic diseases and conditions / Monte Lai, Ph.D., Former Professor of Biophysics,
    Medical College of Wisconsin, USA.
Description: New Jersey : World Scientific, [2020] | Includes bibliographical references and index.
Identifiers: LCCN 2019058296 | ISBN 9789811215247 (hardcover) |
    ISBN 9789811215889 (paperback) | ISBN 9789811215254 (ebook)
Subjects: LCSH: Diet therapy--Popular works. | Diseases--Alternative treatment. |
    Antioxidants--Therapeutic use.
Classification: LCC RM216 .L33 2020 | DDC 615.8/54--dc23
LC record available at https://lccn.loc.gov/2019058296

British Library Cataloguing-in-Publication Data
A catalogue record for this book is available from the British Library.

For any available supplementary material, please visit
https://www.worldscientific.com/worldscibooks/10.1142/11691#t=suppl

Printed in Singapore

For my grandchildren
Olivia, Herbert, Ailann, and Maya

"Let food be thy medicine and medicine be thy food."

Hippocrates (460–370 BCE)
(The father of modern medicine)

Contents

Introduction

In 2019, the United States national health expenditure will reach $4.5 trillion. The medical expenditure is now $13,387 per capita, which is twice as much as that in any other developed country. Overall, 75% of the budget is allocated for the care and management of patients with chronic diseases, such as hypertension, type 2 diabetes, heart disease, Alzheimer's disease, and cancer. With 76.4 million of baby boomers, the national health expenditure will continue skyrocketing and the healthcare system will become unsustainable in the foreseeable future.

It is well known in the medical community that at least 75% of all chronic diseases are preventable by dietary and lifestyle changes. About 74% of all food items in the American grocery stores are processed foods, most of which contain high contents of salt, fat, and/or sugar. Habitual consumption of processed foods and fast foods, which lack essential vitamins and nutrients, such as omega-3 fatty acids and dietary fiber, can cause nutrient and vitamin insufficiencies, resulting in obesity and insulin resistance. About one half of all American adults are overweight and one third are obese. Obesity and insulin resistance can lead to a host of chronic disease, including hypertension, type 2 diabetes, Alzheimer's disease, and cancer.

In addition, the habitual consumption of processed foods and fast foods, which are low in antioxidant contents, can bring on oxidative stress, mediated by excessive free radicals (molecules with unpaired electrons). The symptoms of oxidative stress include grey hair, wrinkles, diminished eye sight, fatigue, memory loss, muscle and/or joint pain, and susceptibility to infections. In severe cases, oxidative stress can lead to diabetes, neurodegenerative diseases, inflammation, cardiovascular disease, and aging.

As an example, for oxidative stress, monosaccharides, such as glucose, can bind to hemoglobin through a free radical-mediated reaction and form a glycated hemoglobin or hemoglobin A1c, an adduct that alters hemoglobin structure and renders it useless. Imagine that an army of glucose attacks hemoglobin molecules in red blood cells and destroys red blood cells that carry oxygen. This scenario replays itself daily in patients with type 2 diabetes. Glucose not only can destroy hemoglobin molecules, it can also destroy other proteins that line the capillary beds, particularly in the extremities. Severe diabetic patients often require amputation of ulcerative toes due in part to the destruction of the endothelial proteins in the capillaries caused by high blood glucose.

Another food related free-radical story is nitric oxide, a gaseous free radical that exists in the human body. In 1998, three American scientists received the Nobel Prize in Physiology or Medicine for their co-discovery of nitric oxide and its significance to human health. In the human body, nitric oxide is a strong vasodilator, with a half-life of less than 15 seconds, so it disappears as quickly as it is produced. Because it disappears so quickly, it escaped detection for years. In 1992, when I was a professor at the Medical College of Wisconsin, I demonstrated for the first time in history the existence of nitric oxide in a live animal experiment using Electron Spin Resonance spectroscopy. Discovering the existence of nitric oxide in the human body drew my attention to the safety of nitrites and nitrates, which are commonly used meat preservatives. During meat curing and preserving process, nitrites release nitric oxide, which binds to the heme of the hemoglobin molecule and forms nitrosyl-hemoglobin. Bacteria need iron to grow and multiply, but they cannot utilize the iron in nitrosyl-hemoglobin. Without iron, bacteria cannot survive. That is why sausages and hotdogs can be kept at ambient temperature for a very long period. When I learned that, I decided to quit eating sausages and other processed meat, since they are foods that even bacteria do not care to eat.

There are three ways to change dietary habits. First, cook at home and avoid eating out. When you cook at home, you know exactly what you are eating. When eating in a restaurant, you cannot be sure what ingredients are in your food. Second, eat more fruits, vegetables, whole grains, nuts, fish, olive oil, and dairy foods. Third, avoid red meat, processed meat, sugar-sweetened beverages, artificial sweetener beverages, and salty foods.

In my first book, *The Vitamin Cure: Clinically Proven Remedies to Prevent and Treat 75 Chronic Diseases and Conditions*, I introduced readers to the concept of correctly using vitamins and essential elements to prevent and treat chronic diseases. All the data presented in that book came from meta-analytic papers published in hundreds of peer-reviewed scientific journals. Meta-analysis is a statistical method that combines data from multiple clinical trials (excluding the data that it deems biased) and analyzes the remainder of the combined data to reach a statistical conclusion. Meta-analysis is currently the most reliable method for assessing the efficacies of vitamins and essential elements in preventing and treating chronic diseases and conditions.

While writing my first book, I came across hundreds of peer-reviewed meta-analysis publications about antioxidant foods in relation to chronic diseases. These meta-analysis publications are the collective work of numerous scientists and physicians who studied the dietary habits of millions of people worldwide and discovered that individuals with nutrient deficiencies benefit from correct food intake, which can restore health and prevent and treat many chronic diseases. This treasure trove of valuable information is scattered and hidden in those published scientific journals and is not accessible to the public. The aim of this book is to provide you with the meta-analytical confirmation that antioxidant-rich foods, such as fruits, vegetables, whole grains, nuts, olive oil, and fish, are clinically proven food remedies that can prevent and treat many chronic diseases, including hypertension, type 2 diabetes, heart disease, stroke, cancers, Alzheimer's disease, and the like.

This book is divided into three parts. Part One presents thirty clinically proven antioxidant foods to prevent and treat chronic diseases. It is comprised of thirty chapters, and each chapter covers an antioxidant food remedy, meta-analytical confirmation of its role in preventing and treating chronic diseases and recommended daily intakes. These thirty antioxidant food remedies are aloe vera, apple, avocado, berries, cheese, cinnamon, cocoa/dark chocolate, citrus fruits, cruciferous vegetables, dietary fiber, fish, flaxseed, fruits, garlic, ginger, grape seed extract, legumes, low salt, milk, nuts, olive oil, pomegranates, probiotics, resveratrol, rice bran oil, soy foods, tomato, vegetables, and whole grains.

Part Two addresses seven disease-causative foods, including red meat, processed meat, sugar-sweetened beverages, artificially-sweetened beverages, high glycemic-load foods, salty foods, and eggs. It contains seven chapters, and each chapter covers the harmful effects of an unhealthy food and meta-analytic confirmation of its role in causing chronic disease.

Part Three identifies twenty-one chronic diseases and their clinically proven antioxidant foods and disease-causative foods. It consists of twenty-one chapters; each chapter discusses one chronic disease, the meta-analytical clinical proof of both corresponding antioxidant foods and of disease-causative foods. These twenty-one chronic diseases are breast cancer, cardiovascular disease, chronic kidney disease, cognitive impairment, colorectal cancer, endometrial cancer, esophageal cancer, heart disease, hypercholesterolemia, hypertension, liver cancer, lung cancer, obesity, oral cancer, ovarian cancer, pancreatic cancer, premature mortality, prostate cancer, stomach cancer, stroke, and type 2 diabetes.

Author's disclaimer: This book provides readers with relevant information about foods to prevent and treat chronic diseases. It is not a substitute for medical advice given to readers by healthcare professionals. The effectiveness of foods in preventing or treating diseases may vary greatly among individuals. Recommendations from the book should not replace any prescribed medication.

Part One

Thirty Clinically Proven Antioxidant Foods to Prevent and Treat Chronic Diseases

Any living organism needs energy to maintain its characteristic shape and form, regulate metabolisms, cope with ever-changing environment. Most importantly, living organisms need energy to reproduce and maintain the existence of the species in perpetuity. Chlorophyll in plants take energy from the Sun's rays and convert it to glucose via a biochemical process called photosynthesis. Plant cells then convert glucose to other biomolecules such as carbohydrates, proteins, lipids, nucleic acids, and a myriad of small cellular molecules. Thus, the energy from the Sun is a necessary condition for the creation of all plant species on Earth. Chlorophyll is an amazing molecule that can capture the energy from the Sun. Animals do not have chlorophyll, so they cannot utilize the Sun's rays to produce energy. To obtain energy, all animals need to consume plants and other animals. Some animals, such as cows, sheep, and elephants, only consume plants, while others, such as tigers and lions only consume other animals. From an evolutionary viewpoint, humans are omnivorous; although we do consume other animals, our main food sources are grains, fruits, and vegetables. Humans derive energy chiefly from plants, not from other animals. We eat other animals to obtain nutrients such as docosahexaenoic acid (DHA), an essential omega-3 fatty acid, which is absent in plants, rather than eat other animals for the bulk of our energy needs.

In the past ten years, researchers have conducted meta-analyses (combined data from multiple studies) to sort through published clinical studies of the dietary habits of millions of people worldwide and have identified thirty antioxidant foods to prevent and treat chronic diseases. These thirty clinically proven food remedies listed in alphabetical order are aloe vera, apple, avocado, berries, cheese, cinnamon, cocoa/dark chocolate, cruciferous vegetables, citrus fruits, dietary fiber, fish, flaxseed, fruits, garlic, ginger, grape seed extract, legumes, low salt, milk, nuts, olive oil, pomegranates, probiotics, resveratrol, rice bran oil, soy foods, tomato, vegetables, and whole grains.

1

Aloe Vera

The aloe vera plant originated in the southwest Arabian Peninsula. Its name is derived from the Arabic word "alloeh", which means bitter. An aloe vera plant can grow to maturity in 3–4 years and reach 30 inches in height with up to 21 leaves; each leaf is about 12–20 inches long and 4 inches broad at the base. The aloe vera plant is grown commercially to extract the juice inside its leaves which has health benefits. About 60–65% of the aloe vera in the world market is produced in the United States.

Recognition of the medicinal benefits of aloe vera dates back as far as 4,000 years ago in ancient Egypt. The nourishing juice of the aloe vera plant was used to treat burns, infection, inflammation, wound healing, and reduce fever. Legend has it that Cleopatra used aloe vera for her skin care and beauty regime. Alexander the Great heeded the advice of Aristotle to capture the Island of Socotra off the coast of Africa, at that time the center of aloe vera production, to acquire enough supplies of aloe vera for healing the wounds of his warriors.

Aloe vera contains at least 75 bioactive compounds including antioxidant vitamins, essential elements, and phytochemicals, such as anthraquinone, anthrones, and glucomannan. Glucomannan is known to reduce blood glucose level, ameliorate inflammation, and support immune function. In addition, anthraquinone and anthrones can increase insulin sensitivity, stimulate the pancreas to produce insulin, regulate the metabolism of glucose, and reduce the risk of type 2 diabetes.

What Types of Chronic Disease can be Prevented by Consuming Aloe Vera Juice?

• Meta-analysis

Type 2 diabetes — Aloe vera juice intake lowers fasting glucose and hemoglobin A1c levels in type 2 diabetic patients as well as fasting glucose level in pre-diabetic individuals.

A meta-analysis examined the association between aloe vera juice intake and type 2 diabetes found that type 2 diabetic patients who regularly consumed aloe vera juice decreased fasting glucose level by 21.3 mg/dL and HbA1c by 1.1%, and pre-diabetic individuals who regularly consumed aloe vera juice decreased fasting glucose level by 4.0 mg/dL.

• Conclusion

Aloe vera juice intake has a favorable influence on glycemic control in patients with type 2 diabetes as well as in pre-diabetic individuals (see Table 1.1). Aloe vera juice should be included in a healthy diet to prevent and treat type 2 diabetes.

Table 1.1. Meta-analytical Confirmation of Aloe Vera Juice Intake Associated with a Lower Risk of Type 2 Diabetes

Chronic Diseases	Reduced Risk, Aloe Vera Juice
Type 2 diabetes	Aloe vera juice reduced fasting glucose level by 4 mg/dL in prediabetic individuals. Aloe vera juice reduced fasting glucose level by 21.1 mg/dL and HbA1c by 1.1% in patients with type 2 diabetes.

- # Recommendation

Prevention — For people at risk of type 2 diabetes: the recommended dose for men is 1 teaspoon of aloe vera juice twice per day, and the recommended dose for women is ½ teaspoon of aloe vera juice twice per day.

Treatment — For type 2 diabetic patients: the recommended dose for men is 1 teaspoon of aloe vera juice three times per day, and the recommended dose for women is ½ teaspoon of aloe vera three times per day.

Material: Select organic aloe vera juice with no preservatives. Some aloe vera products are for external uses, such as for hair care and skin care purposes. When purchasing, make sure that the product is not for external use. In addition to aloe vera juice supplements, aloe vera gel capsules are also available in the marketplace. You may also purchase organic aloe vera powder and reconstitute it with water to make pure aloe vera juice at home. Typically, 1 portion of aloe vera powder is added to 99 portions of water to produce pure aloe vera juice. Aloe vera juice should be placed in the refrigerator to preserve its freshness.

2

Apple

In ancient times, apples already were a favored fruit. The four oldest civilizations of the world, China, Egypt, Greece, and Roman, all had well-kept, detailed records of local apple production, including the variety, tastes, size, and scale of apple orchards. In the 1st century, there were only 23 different kinds of apples. Currently, there are more than 5,000 varieties of apples available in the world.

Apples contain concentrated amounts of polyphenolic compounds, which account for the color, taste, flavor, and health benefits to humans. Polyphenolic compounds can quench free radicals and reduce the risk of oxidative stress, which is known to play a role in the pathogenesis of chronic diseases. Furthermore, polyphenolic compounds such as phloridzin can attenuate several disease-related processes, including inflammation, cell proliferation, and tumor formation.

People living in Wales in 1922 propagated the adage about the benefits of daily apple consumption: "An apple a day keeps the doctor away." Without any supporting evidence, the Welsh ascertained the health benefits of apple consumption in the 1920s. Can it be true that people who eat apples have a lower risk of suffering from chronic diseases?

What Types of Chronic Disease can be Prevented by Consuming Apples?

• Meta-analysis

Breast cancer — Women who regularly consume apples have lower risk of breast cancer.

Eight research papers evaluating the relationship between apple consumption and breast cancer reported that regular consumption of apples decreased the risk of breast cancer by 21% in pre- and postmenopausal women.

Colorectal cancer — Apple consumption can significantly lower the risk of colorectal cancer.

A meta-analysis of five research papers showed that apple consumption reduced the risk of colorectal cancer by 34%.

Lung cancer — Apple consumption greatly reduces the risk of lung cancer.

Ten clinical reports evaluated the relationship between apple intake and lung cancer found that consumption of apples reduced the risk of lung cancer by 18%.

Obesity — Daily consumption of apples can lead to weight loss and a lower risk of obesity.

A meta-analysis of three prospective studies in 133,468 people revealed that each additional serving of apple daily reduced 1.24 lbs in weight.

Type 2 diabetes — People who consume apples daily have a lower risk of type 2 diabetes.

Five prospective studies explored the relationship between apple consumption and type 2 diabetes in 228,315 people. The analysis revealed that consuming apples daily reduced the risk of type 2 diabetes by 18%. In addition, each additional serving of apple per week curtailed the risk of type 2 diabetes by 3%.

• Conclusion

The meta-analytical data has shown that apple consumption lowered body weight and reduced the risk of type 2 diabetes, lung cancer, breast cancer, and colorectal cancer. Pre-diabetic individuals who consumed apples daily reduced their weight by 1.24 lbs and lowered their risk of type 2 diabetes by 18%. In addition, consuming apples daily reduced the risk of lung cancer, breast cancer, and colorectal cancer by 18%, 21%, and 34%, respectively.

In summary, apple consumption can promote weight loss and reduce the risk of type 2 diabetes in prediabetic patients. In addition, daily consumption of apples is associated with lower risks of lung cancer, colorectal cancer, and breast cancer. Apples should be included in the dietary recommendations for the prevention and management of chronic diseases.

Table 2.1. Meta-analytical Confirmation of Apple Intake Associated with Lower Risk of Chronic Diseases

Chronic Diseases	Reduced Risk, Apples
Breast cancer	Apples reduced the risk of breast cancer by 21%.
Colorectal cancer	Apples reduced the risk of colorectal cancer by 34%.
Lung cancer	Apples reduced the risk of lung cancer by 18%.
Obesity	Each additional serving of apples per day reduced weight by 1.24 lbs.
Type 2 diabetes	Apples reduced the risk of type 2 diabetes by18%. Each additional serving of apples per week reduced the risk of type 2 diabetes by 3%.

• Recommendation

Prevention — For people at risk of chronic diseases: men should consume 1 apple per day, and women should consume one apple per day.

Treatment — For chronic disease patients: men should consume ½ apple three times per day, and women should consume one apple per day.

Material: A variety of apples is available in the marketplace. Select your own favorites. One mid-size apple is about 70–100 grams.

3

Avocado

Avocados are native to Central America. Avocado was called, "ahuacati", which means "testicle" in the Aztec language. According to archeological records, avocado had become a staple food of the aboriginal Mexicans by 10,000 BCE. Avocado was first brought to the US grocery stores in the 19th century. Initially, people who lived in California, Florida, and Hawaii liked the taste of avocado, but the rest of the country did not seem to care for it. In the 1950s, avocado slices added to fresh salad plates gained acceptance, and the Americans have since then developed a tasty palate for avocado. Now avocados can be found in grocery stores across the country.

Avocados are rich in lycopene and beta-carotene, both of which belong to antioxidant carotenoids. The dark green flesh closest to the peel in fresh avocados contains the highest concentration of these antioxidant carotenoids. Avocados also contain abundant amounts of plant oils, including 71% monounsaturated fatty acids, 13% polyunsaturated fatty acids, and 16% saturated fatty acids, as well as high amounts of nutrients, such as potassium, magnesium, B vitamins, Vitamin E, Vitamin K, dietary fiber, and lignans.

What Types of Chronic Disease can be Prevented by Consuming Avocados?

• Meta-analysis

Hypercholesterolemia — Daily consumption of avocados significantly lowers blood cholesterol levels and improves blood lipid profiles in hypercholesterolemic patients.

A meta-analysis of ten double-blind randomized clinical trials investigated the relationship between avocados and hypercholesterolemia found that daily consumption of avocados decreased total cholesterol level by 18.8 mg/dL, LDL cholesterol level by 16.5 mg/dL, and triglycerides by 27.20 mg/dL in hypercholesterolemic patients.

• Conclusion

Daily consumption of avocados decreased the total cholesterol level, LDL cholesterol level, and triglycerides in hypercholesterolemic patients as shown in Table 3.1. The results support the notion that consuming avocados can favorably improve blood lipids and lipoproteins in patients with hypercholesterolemia. The extent to which blood cholesterol levels reduced by avocados resembles that observed by anti-cholesterol medications. Adding avocado to a healthy diet can improve blood lipid profiles as well as mitigate the condition of the disease in patients with hypercholesterolemia. Avocados should be included in the

Table 3.1. Meta-analytical Confirmation of Avocado Consumption Associated with a Lower Risk of Hypercholesterolemia

Chronic Diseases	Reduced Risk, Avocados
Hypercholesterolemia	Avocados decreased total cholesterol level by 19 mg/dL, LDL cholesterol level by17 mg/dL, and triglycerides by 27 mg/dL in hypercholesterolemic patients.

dietary recommendations for the prevention and the management of hypercholesterolemia.

• Recommendation

Prevention — For people at risk of hypercholesterolemia: men should consume 1 mid-size avocado each day, and women should consume ½ of a mid-size avocado each day.

Treatment — For hypercholesterolemic patients: men should consume 1½ of mid-size avocados each day, and women should consume 1 mid-size avocado per day.

Materials: Avocados produced in California on average weigh about 6 ounces (or 170 g) each. Place avocados at ambient temperature until they are almost ripened and then store them in the refrigerator to slow down ripening process and preserve their freshness.

4

Berries

For thousands of years, berries were a seasonal staple for hunter-gatherers, and to this date, wild berry gathering is still a popular activity in Europe and North America. Blueberries originated in North America. They were gathered and used by the native Americans for centuries. The United States is now the leading country in blueberry production, and it supplies about 90% of all blueberries in the world market. Strawberries, which belong to the rose family, are also native to North America. Cultivation of strawberries started in the 19th century in the United States, and about 75% of all strawberries in the United States are now produced in California.

Berries contain high amounts of polyphenols, including anthocyanins, proanthocyanidins, quercetin, and phenolic acid. These phytochemicals, particularly anthocyanins, can inhibit lymphocytes from producing free radicals and prevent the oxidation of LDL cholesterol. Anti-inflammatory anthocyanins can also inhibit atherosclerosis and prevent cardiovascular diseases.

What Types of Chronic Disease can be Prevented by Consuming Berries?

• Meta-analysis

Cardiovascular disease — Berry consumption reduces blood cholesterol, blood pressure, and fasting glucose levels and mitigates the condition of the disease in patients with cardiovascular disease.

Twenty-two double-blind randomized clinical trials studied the association between berry consumption and cardiovascular disease. The meta-analysis results showed that berry consumption (primarily blueberries and cranberries) decreased LDL cholesterol level by 3.8 mg/dL, systolic pressure by 2.73 mmHg, and fasting glucose levels by 1.8 mg/dL in cardiovascular disease patients. Berry intake was also found to reduce body mass index, hemoglobin A1c, and tumor necrosis factor-alpha.

• Conclusion

Berry consumption, as evidenced from the meta-analytical results, reduced LDL cholesterol level by 4 mg/dL, systolic pressure by 3 mmHg, and fasting glucose level by 2 mg/dL in patients with cardiovascular disease, as shown in Table 4.1. The results are consistent with the view that berry consumption can lower blood cholesterol, blood pressure, and fasting glucose levels, all of which are risk factors of cardiovascular disease. Berries, including blueberries and strawberries, should be included in a healthy diet to prevent and treat cardiovascular disease.

Table 4.1. Meta-analytical Confirmation of Berry Consumption Associated with a Lower Risk of Cardiovascular Disease

Chronic Disease	Reduced Risk, Berries
Cardiovascular disease	Berries decreased LDL cholesterol level by 3.8 mg/dL, systolic pressure by 3 mmHg and fasting glucose by 2 mg/dL in cardiovascular disease patients.

• Recommendation

Prevention — For people at risk of cardiovascular disease: consume ¼ cup of mixed berries per day.

Treatment — For cardiovascular disease patients: consume ½ cup of mixed berries per day.

Materials: When choosing berries, select blueberries, cranberries, strawberries, and the like.

5

Cheese

During the Agriculture Era, humans domesticated milk producing animals, particularly sheep, and produced cheese, although the exact origin of cheese and cheese making is not known. Cheese may have been produced accidentally by storing milk in containers made from animal stomachs, by salting milk for preservation purposes, or by adding fruit juices to milk, each of which would cause the milk to coagulate and form curds. By Roman times, cheese became popular, and the cheese making techniques quickly spread to the Middle East and throughout Europe.

During the fermentation process, proteins in milk are broken down to produce antioxidant peptides, which can reduce oxidative stress and protect against chronic diseases, such as type 2 diabetes. These antioxidant peptides also contribute to favorable influences in modulating cholesterol synthesis in the liver and reducing total cholesterol and LDL cholesterol levels in the bloodstream.

What Types of Chronic Disease can be Prevented by Consuming Cheese?

• Meta-analysis

Hypercholesterolemia — Cheese consumption lowers blood cholesterol levels and improves lipoprotein profiles in patients with cholesterolemia.

Twelve double-blind randomized clinical trials investigated the relationship between cheese consumption and hypercholesterolemia found that daily consumption of 145 g of cheese decreased LDL cholesterol level by 6.5% and increased HDL cholesterol level by 3.9% in patients with hypercholesterolemia.

Type 2 diabetes — Daily consumption of cheese can reduce the risk of type 2 diabetes.

Fourteen prospective studies investigated the association between cheese consumption and type 2 diabetes in 426,055 people showed that daily intake of 50 g of cheese reduced the risk of type 2 diabetes by 8%.

• Conclusion

Cheese consumption decreased the LDL cholesterol level and increase HDL cholesterol level in patients with hypercholesterolemia and reduced the risk of type 2 diabetes in pre-diabetic individuals. A daily consumption of 5 ounces of cheese decreased the LDL cholesterol level by 6.5% and increased the HDL cholesterol level by 3.5% in patients with high blood cholesterol level. In addition, a daily consumption of 2 ounces of cheese reduced the risk of type 2 diabetes by 8% as shown in Table 5.1. Adding cheese to a nutrient-balanced diet can favorably improve blood lipid profiles in patients with hypercholesterolemia as well as reduce the risk of type 2 diabetes in prediabetic individuals.

Table 5.1. Meta-analytical Confirmation of Cheese Consumption Associated with Lower Risks of Hypercholesterolemia and Type 2 Diabetes

Chronic Disease	Reduced Risk, Cheese
Hypercholesterolemia	Daily intake of 5 ounces of cheese decreased LDL cholesterol level by 6.5% and increased HDL cholesterol level by 3.5% in hypercholesterolemic patients.
Type 2 diabetes	Daily intake of 2 ounces of cheese reduced the risk of type 2 diabetes by 8%.

- ## Recommendation

Prevention — For people at risk of hypercholesterolemia: men should consume one ounce of cheese per day, and women should consume ½ ounce of cheese per day.

Treatment — For hypercholesterolemic patients: men should consume one ounce of cheese twice per day, and women should consume ½ ounce of cheese twice per day.

Materials: Great varieties of cheese products are available in the marketplace. Select your favorite cheese and enjoy them alone or with meals.

6

Cinnamon

The cinnamon tree originated in Ceylon, the present-day Sri Lanka. In 1518, Portuguese sailors invaded the island Kingdom of Kotto and gained control of the cinnamon trade for over a century. The cinnamon trade in Sri Lanka was handed over to the Dutch in the 17th century and then to the British in the 18th century. During that period, cinnamon was considered a rare and expensive spice enjoyed only by the riches and nobles in the world. By 1800, cinnamon was vastly cultivated in many parts of the world, and its price precipitously dropped and became within the reach of common people.

Since ancient times, humans have recognized the medicinal benefits of cinnamon. The bark, leaves, flowers, fruits, and roots of cinnamon trees all have condimental or medicinal value. Cinnamon powder derived from the bark of cinnamon tree contains high amounts of dietary fiber and polyphenols, both of which can slow down the absorption of cholesterol and fats by the intestines, decrease blood cholesterol level, and improve blood lipid profile. In addition, the polyphenols in cinnamon are known antioxidants, which can enhance anti-inflammatory functions to prevent type 2 diabetes.

What Types of Chronic Disease can be Prevented by Consuming Cinnamon?

- ## Meta-analysis

Hypercholesterolemia — Cinnamon powder intake lowers blood cholesterol levels and improves blood lipid profiles in patients with cholesterolemia.

Ten randomized controlled trials investigated the relationship between cinnamon intake and hypercholesterolemia found that a daily consumption of 120 mg of cinnamon powder for 4–18 weeks decreased total cholesterol level by 15.6 mg/dL, LDL cholesterol level by 9.42 mg/dL and triglycerides by 29.59 mg/dL, while it increased HDL cholesterol level by 1.66 mg/dL in hypercholesterolemic patients.

Type 2 diabetes — Intake of cinnamon powder significantly lowers the fasting glucose level in patients with type 2 diabetes.

A meta-analysis of six randomized controlled trials explored the association between cinnamon intake and the risk of type 2 diabetes revealed that a daily intake of 1–6 g of cinnamon for 40 days to 4 months reduced the fasting glucose level by 15.3 mg/dL and HbA1c value by 0.09% in type 2 diabetic patients, which suggests that cinnamon intake can mitigate the condition of the disease in type 2 diabetic patients. Another meta-analysis of ten randomized controlled trials examined the relationship between cinnamon intake and the risk of type 2 diabetes found that a daily intake of 120 mg of cinnamon powder for 4 to 18 weeks reduced the fasting glucose level by 24.6 mg/dL in patients with type 2 diabetes.

- ## Conclusion

A daily intake of cinnamon powder decreased the total cholesterol level by 15.6 mg/dL, LDL cholesterol level by 9.42 mg/dL and triglycerides by 30 mg/dL and increased the HDL cholesterol level by 1.66 mg/dL in patients with hypercholesterolemia (see Table 6.1). In addition, a daily intake of 120 mg of cinnamon powder for 4 to 18 weeks reduced the fasting glucose level by 24.6 mg/dL in type 2 diabetic patients. The results provide compelling evidence that cinnamon powder is effective in improving blood lipid profiles in patients with hypercholesterolemia and in lowering the blood glucose level in patients with type 2 diabetes. Adding cinnamon powder to a healthy diet may prevent hypercholesterolemia and type 2 diabetes, as well as ameliorate the condition of the disease in patients with hypercholesterolemia and patients with type 2 diabetes.

Table 6.1.   Meta-analytical Confirmation of Cinnamon Intake Associated with an Improved Blood Lipid Profiles in Patients with Hypercholesterolemia

Chronic Disease	Reduced Risk, Cinnamon Intake
Hypercholesterolemia	Daily intake of 120 mg of cinnamon powder for 4–18 weeks decreased total cholesterol level by 15.6 mg/dL, LDL cholesterol level by 9.42 mg/dL, triglycerides by 30 mg/dL, and increased HDL cholesterol level by 1.66 mg/dL in patients with hypercholesterolemia.
Type 2 diabetes	Intake of 120 mg of cinnamon powder daily for 4–18 weeks reduced fasting glucose level by 24.6 mg/dL in type 2 diabetic patients.
	Daily consumption of 1–6 g of cinnamon for 40 days to 4 months reduced fasting glucose level by 15.3 mg/dL and HbA1c value by 0.09% in patients with type 2 diabetes.

• **Recommendation**

Prevention — For people at risk of hypercholesterolemia and type 2 diabetes: the recommended dose for men is ½ teaspoon of cinnamon powder per day, and the recommended dose for women is ¼ teaspoon of cinnamon powder a day.

Treatment — For hypercholesterolemia and type 2 diabetic patients: the recommended dose for men is one teaspoon of cinnamon powder per day, and the recommended dose for women is ½ teaspoon of cinnamon powder per day.

Materials: In the marketplace, cinnamon powder mainly comes from two different sources, Chinese cinnamon and Ceylonese cinnamon. Chinese cinnamon or also known as Saigon cinnamon contains a high amount of coumadin. The side effects of coumadin include delayed wound healing and liver toxicity. When purchasing, select Ceylonese cinnamon, not Chinese cinnamon or Saigon cinnamon. Cinnamon powder can be added to your favorite meals.

7

Citrus Fruits

Orange is a native plant of India. Archeological records have revealed that in 7000 BCE, Indians domesticated orange trees. To this date, orange peel and orange juice are still used as ingredients in some Indian-style cooking and dishes. Around 500 BCE, orange cultivation spread to China, and wealthy and noble families during Zhou Dynasty loved to brag about the size of their orange orchards and the taste of their oranges. In Roman times, only nobles could afford expensive oranges imported from India. The Romans soon grew their own oranges in North Africa. In the 16th century, the Spaniards occupied Florida and operated large-scale orange orchards there. Florida is now the second largest orange producing region in the world.

In 1753, James Lind demonstrated experimentally that sailors who consumed citrus fruits during long sea voyages were spared from scurvy. In 1928, Albert Szent-Gyorgyi discovered that scurvy was caused by Vitamin C deficiency and Vitamin C alone cured scurvy disease. Owing to his discovery of Vitamin C and contributions to medicine, Szent-Gyorgyi was awarded the 1937 Nobel Prize in Physiology or Medicine. Besides antioxidant Vitamin C, citrus fruits, such as oranges, also are good sources of potassium, calcium, copper, and magnesium, and B vitamins, including Vitamin B1, Vitamin B2, Vitamin B3, Vitamin B5, Vitamin B6, and Vitamin B9.

What Types of Chronic Disease can be Prevented by Consuming Citrus Fruits?

• Meta-analysis

Breast cancer — Women who regularly consume citrus fruits have a lower risk of breast cancer.

Six research papers investigated the relationship between citrus fruit intake and breast cancer in 8,393 women found that regular consumption of citrus fruits reduced the risk of breast cancer by 13%.

Esophageal cancer — Citrus fruit intake reduces the risk of esophageal cancer.

A meta-analysis of 13 case-control studies and six prospective studies examined the association between citrus fruit consumption and esophageal cancer showed that consumption of citrus fruits reduced the risk of esophageal cancer by 37%.

Pancreatic cancer — Frequent consumption of citrus fruits lowers the risk of pancreatic cancer.

A meta-analysis of nine research papers investigated the association between citrus fruit intake and pancreatic cancer found that intake of citrus fruits reduced the risk of pancreatic cancer by 17%.

Stomach cancer — High consumption of citrus fruits greatly reduces the risk of stomach cancer.

Five research articles evaluated the relationship between citrus fruit consumption and stomach cancer in 1,286,930 people including 2,324 gastric cancer cases. The analysis showed that high consumption of citrus fruits reduced the risk of stomach cancer by 13%. The dose-response analysis revealed that each additional intake of 100 g of citrus fruits per day reduced the risk of stomach cancer by 40%.

• Conclusion

Table 7.1 illustrates that consumption of citrus fruits reduced the risk of breast cancer, esophageal cancer, stomach cancer, and pancreatic cancer. People who consumed citrus fruits daily reduced the risk of esophageal cancer, stomach cancer, and pancreatic cancer by 37%, 40%, and 17%, respectively. In addition, a daily intake of 100 g of citrus fruits reduced the risk of stomach cancer by 40%. Moreover, women who consumed citrus fruits reduced the risk of breast cancer by 10%.

In summary, the intake of citrus fruits is associated with lower risks of cancers, including esophageal cancer, stomach cancer, pancreatic cancer, and breast cancer. Citrus fruits should be included as part of a healthy diet for the prevention and management of cancers.

Table 7.1. Meta-analytical Confirmation of Intake of Citrus Fruits Associated with Lower Risks of Chronic Diseases

Chronic Diseases	Reduced Risk, Citrus Fruits
Breast cancer	Citrus fruits reduced the risk of breast cancer by 10%.
Esophageal cancer	Citrus fruits reduced the risk of esophageal cancer by 37%.
Pancreatic cancer	Citrus fruits reduced the risk of pancreatic cancer by 17%.
Stomach cancer	Citrus fruits reduced the risk of stomach cancer by 13%.

• Recommendation

Prevention — For people at risk of chronic diseases: men should consume 1 mid-size orange or tangerine per day, and women should consume 1 mid-size orange or tangerine per day.

Treatment — For chronic disease patients: men should consume 1 mid-size orange or tangerine, twice per day, and women should consume ½ mid-size orange or tangerine, three times per day.

Material: According to USDA data, one large orange is about 184 g and one mid-size orange is about 131 g.

Are the naturally present sugars in fruits harmful to health?

Natural sugars such as fructose and sucrose are found in fruits. Fructose is harmful only if it is consumed in large amounts, such as in sugar-sweetened beverages. It is not possible to consume a large amount of fructose by eating fruits. Besides, fruits are excellent sources of dietary fiber, which can obstruct the small intestines' absorption of fructose. In other words, only a portion of fructose in fruits is absorbed by the small intestines, while almost 100% of fructose in sugar-sweetened beverage is absorbed by the small intestines. Furthermore, fruits contain many other nutrients, such as antioxidant vitamins and essential elements, whereas sugar-sweetened beverages contain no such nutrients. Fructose and other natural sugars present in fruits are harmless, and it is safe to enjoy fruits.

8

Cocoa Products/Dark Chocolate

The cocoa tree is a native of the Yucatan Peninsula, a tropical area of southern Mexico, where the Mayan people first discovered the delicious, healthy cocoa food around 600 CE. In the 16th century, the Spaniards invaded Mexico and kept the secret of cocoa beans to themselves for a century. By the mid-17th century, Spain lost its control of the European chocolate market, and cocoa beans soon became popular in France and other European countries. Both cocoa products and dark chocolate are favorite foods among people of all age groups. Globally, the annual consumption of cocoa beans is estimated to be more than 4.5 million tons. Americans, on average, consume about 5 kg of chocolate per capita per year.

Cocoa products and dark chocolate contain abundant amounts of polyphenols, which can scavenge free radicals, inhibit the intestines' absorption of cholesterol, reduce cholesterol synthesis in the liver, and favorably affect blood lipids and lipoproteins.

What Types of Chronic Disease can be Prevented by Consuming Cocoa Products/Dark Chocolate?

• Meta-analysis

Hypercholesterolemia — Regular consumption of cocoa products/ dark chocolate reduces blood cholesterol levels and improves blood lipid profiles in hypercholesterolemic patients.

Ten double-blind randomized clinical trials studied the relationship between cocoa products/dark chocolate and hypercholesterolemia found that consumption of cocoa products/dark chocolate decreased the total cholesterol level by 6.2 mg/dL and LDL cholesterol level by 5.9 mg/dL, but had no discernible effect on HDL cholesterol or triglyceride levels in patients with hypercholesterolemia.

• Conclusion

Consumption of cocoa products and/or dark chocolate favorably decreased total cholesterol and LDL cholesterol levels in patients with hypercholesterolemia. As shown in Table 8.1, consumption of cocoa products and/or dark chocolate decreased the total cholesterol level by 6.2 mg/dL and LDL cholesterol level by 5.9 mg/dL in patients with hypercholesterolemia. The results provide strong evidence that cocoa products and dark chocolate can improve blood lipids and lipoproteins in patients with hypercholesterolemia and should be considered safe and effective food remedies for the prevention and treatment of hypercholesterolemia.

Table 8.1. Meta-analytical Confirmation of Consumption of Cocoa Products/ Dark Chocolate Associated with an Improvement in Blood Lipid Profiles in Patients with Hypercholesterolemia

Chronic Disease	Reduced Risk, Cocoa Products/Dark Chocolate
Hypercholesterolemia	Cocoa products/dark chocolate decreased total cholesterol level by 6.2 mg/dL and LDL cholesterol level by 5.9 mg/ dL in hypercholesterolemic patients.

• Recommendation

Prevention — For people at risk of hypercholesterolemia: men and women should consume 5 g of dark chocolate per day.

Treatment — For hypercholesterolemic patients: men and women should consume 10 g of dark chocolate per day.

Materials: When purchasing, select dark chocolate with no added vegetable oil or sugar. Avoid consuming more than 20 g of dark chocolate a day, because excessive intake of polyphenols from dark chocolate can damage the liver.

9

Cruciferous Vegetables

Cruciferous vegetables include broccoli, cabbage, cauliflower, and kale. Broccoli belongs to cabbage family. Before the Common Era, Tuscany was the agriculture center in Italy. Broccoli was a new species that Tuscan farmers successfully cultivated from cabbage. It had a peculiar taste, but it nevertheless was a favorite food of people during Roman times. Cultivation of broccoli spread from the Mediterranean region to Europe and North America in the mid-18th century, with limited consumer acceptance. During the 1920s, new Italian immigrants brought their home recipes for cooking broccoli to the American soil. Americans embraced the new Italian style of broccoli cuisine. Now, broccoli (either raw or cooked) has become a popular food item in the United States.

Cruciferous vegetables contain a high amount of glucosinolate glucoraphaninan, which can be converted to anti-cancer sulforaphane in the body. Sulforaphane protects against cancer by inactivating carcinogens, enhancing antioxidant, anti-infective, and anti-inflammatory functions, and inhibiting the migration of cancerous cells as well as the formation of new blood vessels in tumor masses.

What Chronic Diseases can be Prevented by Consuming Cruciferous Vegetables?

• Meta-analysis

Breast cancer — Women who regularly consume cruciferous vegetables have lower risk of breast cancer.

A meta-analysis of eleven research papers studied the association between cruciferous vegetable intake and breast cancer showed that consumption of cruciferous vegetables decreased the risk of breast cancer by 15%.

Colorectal cancer — Frequent consumption of cruciferous vegetables lessens the risk of colorectal cancer.

Thirty-three clinical trial reports evaluated the relationship between cruciferous vegetable consumption and colorectal cancer found that consumption of cruciferous vegetables reduced the risk of colorectal cancer by 16%, and consumption of broccoli reduced the risk of colorectal cancer by 20%.

Endometrial cancer — Women who consume cruciferous vegetables (four ounces daily) have lower risks of endometrial cancer.

Seventeen research papers investigated the relationship between cruciferous vegetable consumption and endometrial cancer revealed that women who regularly consumed cruciferous vegetables reduced the risk of endometrial cancer by 15%. The dose-response studies revealed that daily consumption of 100 g of cruciferous vegetables reduced the risk of endometrial cancer by 21%.

Lung cancer — High consumption of cruciferous vegetables curtails the risk of lung cancer, particularly in non-smoking women.

A meta-analysis studied the relationship between cruciferous vegetables and lung cancer in 74,914 women found that women who habitually consumed cruciferous vegetables reduced the risk of lung cancer by 27%, and non-smoking women who habitually consumed cruciferous vegetables reduced the risk of lung cancer by 41%.

Obesity — People who regularly consume cruciferous vegetables lose weight and have lower risks of obesity.

Three research papers evaluated the association between cruciferous vegetable consumption and obesity in 133,468 people revealed that each additional serving of cruciferous vegetables daily reduced body weight by 1.37 lbs.

Ovarian cancer — Women who regularly consume cruciferous vegetables have lower risk of ovarian cancer.

A meta-analysis of eleven research papers investigated the relationship between cruciferous vegetables and ovarian cancer in 375,562 people found that consumption of cruciferous vegetables reduced the risk of ovarian cancer by 16% in pre and postmenopausal women.

Pancreatic cancer — Frequent consumption of cruciferous vegetables significantly decreases the risk of pancreatic cancer.

Nine research papers explored the association between cruciferous vegetable intake and pancreatic cancer revealed that frequent intake of cruciferous vegetables reduced the risk of pancreatic cancer by 22%.

Prostate cancer — Elderly men who regularly consume cruciferous vegetables have lower incidence rates of prostate cancer.

A meta-analysis of 13 research articles studied the relationship between cruciferous vegetable intake and prostate cancer found that consumption of cruciferous vegetables reduced the risk of prostate cancer by 10%.

Stomach cancer — Regular consumption of cruciferous vegetables brings down the risk of stomach cancer.

Twelve research articles evaluated the association between cruciferous vegetables and stomach cancer showed that consumption of cruciferous vegetables reduced the risk of stomach cancer by 19%.

Type 2 diabetes — People who frequently consume cruciferous vegetables have lower risk of type 2 diabetes.

A meta-analysis of 23 research papers investigated the relationship between cruciferous vegetable consumption and type 2 diabetes revealed that cruciferous vegetable consumption reduced the risk of type 2 diabetes by 28%.

• Conclusion

As shown in Table 9.1, obese or overweight individuals who consumed cruciferous vegetables lost about 1.37 lbs on average. In addition, consuming cruciferous vegetables reduced the risk of type 2 diabetes by 38%. Moreover, consumption of cruciferous vegetables reduced the risk of breast cancer, colorectal cancer, and lung cancer by 15%, 16%, and 27%, respectively. In addition, consumption of cruciferous vegetables reduced the risk of ovarian cancer, pancreatic cancer, prostate cancer, and stomach cancer by 16%, 22%, 10%, and 19%, respectively.

The meta-analytical results have demonstrated that consuming cruciferous vegetables promotes weight loss and reduces the risk of type 2 diabetes, breast cancer, endometrial cancer, ovarian cancer, prostate cancer, lung cancer, pancreatic cancer, and colorectal cancer. It is recommended that cruciferous vegetables, such as broccoli, cabbage, and cauliflower, should be included in the dietary recommendations for the prevention and management of type 2 diabetes and cancers.

Table 9.1.   Meta-analytical Confirmation of Cruciferous Vegetables Associated with Lower Risks of Chronic Diseases and Cancers

Chronic Diseases	Reduced Risk, Cruciferous Vegetables
Breast cancer	Cruciferous vegetables reduced the risk of breast cancer by 15%.
Colorectal cancer	Cruciferous vegetables reduced the risk of colorectal cancer by 16%.
Endometrial cancer	Cruciferous vegetables reduced the risk of endometrial cancer by 15%.
Lung cancer	Women who consumed cruciferous vegetables reduced the risk of lung cancer by 27%. Non-smoking women who consumed cruciferous vegetables reduced the risk of lung cancer by 41%.
Obesity	Cruciferous vegetables reduced body weight by 1.37 lbs.
Ovarian cancer	Cruciferous vegetables reduced the risk of ovarian cancer by 16%.

Table 9.1.   (*Continued*)

Chronic Diseases	Reduced Risk, Cruciferous Vegetables
Pancreatic cancer	Cruciferous vegetable reduced the risk of pancreatic cancer by 22%.
Prostate cancer	Cruciferous vegetables reduced the risk of prostate cancer by 22%.
Stomach cancer	Cruciferous vegetables reduced the risk of stomach cancer by 19%.
Type 2 diabetes	Cruciferous vegetables reduced the risk of type 2 diabetes by 38%.

• Recommendation

Prevention — For people at risk of chronic diseases: consume ½ cup of cooked cruciferous vegetables three times per week.

Treatment — For chronic disease patients: consume ½ cup of cooked cruciferous vegetables four times per week.

Materials: Select cruciferous vegetables, such as kale, cabbage, broccoli and cauliflower. Half-cup of cooked broccoli is about 91 grams.

10

Dietary Fiber

Dietary fiber is the collective term of indigestible carbohydrates present in fruits, vegetables, and whole grains. Dietary fibers can be divided into soluble and insoluble, both of which are beneficial to health. Soluble dietary fiber forms a hydrated gel-like substance that helps moisturize the digestive tract. In addition, the beneficial bacteria living in the colon, via the fermentation process, convert soluble dietary fiber to propionic acid and butyric acid. These short-chain fatty acids, particularly butyric acid, can boost the antioxidant defense systems in the body to prevent inflammation and infection, help regulate the cholesterol production in the liver to prevent hypercholesterolemia. Insoluble dietary fiber with high porosity can increase fecal weight, shorten waste retaining time, limit the direct contact of carcinogens with the colon wall, and reduce the risk of colorectal cancer.

What Food Items are Dietary Fiber Rich?

Fruits, vegetables, and whole grains are all excellent sources of dietary fiber. Which food items have higher contents of dietary fiber? Based on the data adapted from the United States Department of Agriculture (USDA), Table 10.1 lists fifteen foods with high dietary fiber contents. Among all vegetables, legumes have the highest amounts of dietary fiber. For example, one cup of cooked lentils

Table 10.1.   Dietary Fiber-rich Food List

Foods	Amount, Intake	Dietary Fiber Content, Grams
Lentils	1 cup, cooked	15.6
Kidney beans	1 cup, cooked	13.6
Prunes	1 cup	12.4
Lima beans	1 cup, cooked	11.6
Peas	1 cup, cooked	8.8
Almonds	½ cup	8.7
Peanuts	½ cup	7.9
Apple	1, mid-size	4.4
Green beans	1 cup, cooked	4.0
Oats	1 cup, cooked	4.0
Potato	1, mid-size	3.8
Brown rice	1 cup, cooked	3.5
Banana	1, mid-size	3.1
Orange	1, mid-size	3.1
Carrots	1 cup, sliced and cooked	2.3

Data adapted from the 2017 USDA sources.

and kidney beans contain 15.6 g and 13.6 g of dietary fiber, respectively, which is equivalent to about one half of the daily recommended fiber intake. Other foods rich in dietary fiber include lima beans, peas, almonds, peanuts, apples, and oats. The United States Institute of Medicine recommends that at age 50 and older men and women should consume 38 g and 25 g of dietary fiber per day, respectively. For people under age 50, daily dietary fiber intake should be 30 g for men and 21 g for women. Currently, the average dietary fiber intake of Americans is about 15 g, which is below the recommended intake levels. Adding foods high in dietary fiber, such as legumes and whole grains, to a healthy diet will help maintain beneficial bacteria flora in the digestive tract and prevent the risk of chronic diseases.

What Types of Chronic Disease can be Prevented by Consuming Foods Rich in Dietary Fiber?

• Meta-analysis

Breast cancer — Women who regularly consume foods rich in dietary fiber have lower risk of breast cancer.

A meta-analysis of twenty-four epidemiological studies investigated the relationship between dietary fiber intake and breast cancer in 3,662,421 people found that consumption of foods rich in dietary fiber reduced the risk of breast cancer by 12%. In addition, daily consumption of 10 g of dietary fiber reduced the risk of breast cancer by 4%.

Cardiovascular disease — Frequent consumption of foods rich in dietary fiber curtails the risk of cardiovascular disease.

Twenty-two prospective studies explored the association between dietary fiber intake and cardiovascular disease showed that each additional intake of 7 g of dietary fiber daily reduced the risk of cardiovascular disease and coronary heart disease by 9% and 9%, respectively.

Chronic kidney disease — Regular consumption of foods rich in dietary fiber lowers serum inflammatory markers and alleviates the condition of the disease in patients with chronic kidney disease.

Fourteen double-blind placebo control clinical trials evaluated the relationship between dietary fiber intake and chronic kidney disease revealed that the intake of dietary fiber reduced serum uric acid level by 1.76 mmol/L and serum creatinine level by 0.42 mg/dL in chronic kidney disease patients.

Colorectal cancer — People who regularly consume foods rich in dietary fiber have lower risk of colorectal cancer.

A meta-analysis of 20 prospective studies investigated the association between dietary fiber intake and colorectal cancer found that consumption of dietary fiber reduced the risk of colorectal cancer by 28%. The dose-response studies revealed that each additional intake of 10 g of dietary fiber per day reduced the risk of colorectal cancer by 9%. When analyzed one by one, fruit dietary fiber, vegetable dietary fiber, and whole grain dietary fiber reduced the risk of colorectal cancer by 16%, 7%, and 24%, respectively.

Endometrial cancer — Women who regularly consume foods rich in dietary fiber have lower risk of endometrial cancer.

Seven research articles explored the relationship between dietary fiber intake and endometrial cancer revealed that consumption of foods rich in dietary fiber reduced the risk of endometrial cancer by 30%. In addition, daily consumption of 5 g of dietary fiber reduced the risk of endometrial cancer by 18% in women on a daily 1,000-calorie diet.

Esophageal cancer — Frequent consumption of foods rich in dietary fiber curtails the risk of esophageal cancer.

Fifteen clinical trial reports investigated the relationship between dietary fiber intake and esophageal cancer in 16,885 people revealed that dietary fiber intake reduced the risk of esophageal cancer by 48%. In addition, each additional intake of 10 g of dietary fiber per day reduced the risk of Barrett's esophagus and esophageal cancer by 31%.

Hypertension — Regular consumption of foods rich in dietary fiber lowers blood pressure in hypertensive patients.

A meta-analysis of 18 double-blind randomized clinical trials studied the association between dietary fiber intake and hypertension found that consuming foods rich in dietary fiber decreased systolic pressure by 0.9 mmHg and diastolic pressure by 0.7 mmHg in hypertensive patients. Additionally, beta-glucan fibers (found in oats and barley) were shown to lower the blood pressure in hypertensive patients.

Pancreatic cancer — High consumption of foods rich in dietary fiber reduces the risk of pancreatic cancer.

Fourteen research reports evaluated the relationship between dietary fiber intake and pancreatic cancer revealed that intake of dietary fiber reduced the risk of pancreatic cancer by 48%. The dose-response analysis revealed that each additional intake of 10 g of dietary fiber per day reduced the risk of pancreatic cancer by 12%.

Premature mortality — People who regularly consume foods rich in dietary fiber have lower risk of premature mortality, including all-cause, cardiovascular disease, coronary heart disease, and cancer mortalities.

A meta-analysis of 17 prospective studies explored the association between dietary fiber intake and premature mortality in 982,411 people, including 67,260 mortality cases showed that dietary fiber intake reduced the risk of all-cause mortality by 16%. The dose-response results indicated that daily intake of 10 g of dietary fiber reduced the risk of all-cause mortality, cardiovascular disease mortality, coronary heart disease mortality, and cancer mortality by 10%, 9%, 11%, and 6%, respectively. In short, a daily intake of dietary fiber can curtail the risk of premature mortality. Another meta-analysis of 15 prospective studies investigated the relationship between dietary fiber intake and premature mortality found that intake of dietary fiber reduced the risk of cardiovascular disease mortality, coronary heart disease mortality, and cancer mortality by 23%, 24%, and 14%, respectively.

Stomach cancer — People who frequently consume foods rich in dietary fiber have lower risk of stomach cancer.

Twenty-one case control studies explored the association between dietary fiber intake and stomach cancer in 580,064 people revealed that high intake of dietary fiber reduced the risk of stomach cancer by 42%. The dose-response studies revealed that each additional intake of 10 g of dietary fiber per day reduced the risk of stomach cancer by 44%.

Stroke — Regular consumption of foods rich in dietary fiber lessens the incidence of stroke, particularly in women.

Six prospective studies investigated the relationship between dietary fiber intake and stroke in 314,864 people including 8,920 stroke cases showed that foods rich in dietary fiber reduced the risk of stroke by 13%. Further studies showed that dietary fiber reduced the risk of stroke by 20% in women and the risk of stroke by 5% in men. Moreover, a daily intake of 10 g of dietary fiber reduced the risk of stroke by 12%.

Type 2 diabetes — High consumption of foods rich in dietary fiber significantly lowers fasting blood glucose levels and favorably improves the condition of the disease in patients with type 2 diabetes.

Eighteen prospective studies investigated the association between dietary fiber intake and type 2 diabetes in 617,968 people including 41,066 type 2 diabetic patients, found that consumption of whole grain dietary fiber, fruit dietary fiber, and vegetable dietary fiber reduced the risk of type 2 diabetes by 25%, 5% and 7%, respectively. In brief, people who consume foods rich in dietary fiber are found to have lower risks of type 2 diabetes. Another meta-analysis of eleven double-blind randomized clinical trials studied the relationship between dietary fiber intake and type 2 diabetes reported that consuming foods rich in dietary fiber decreased the fasting glucose level by 9.97 mg/dL and HbA1c value by 0.55% in type 2 diabetic patients. Analysis confirms that consuming foods rich in dietary fiber improves glycemic control in type 2 diabetic patients. Further supporting evidence about the benefits of dietary fiber, a meta-analysis of 15 double-blind randomized clinical trials showed that consumption of dietary fiber supplement decreased the fasting glucose level by 15.5 mg/dL and HbA1c by 0.26% in type 2 diabetic patients.

• Conclusion

The meta-analytical evidence showed that consumption of dietary fiber reduced the risk of eleven chronic diseases as well as premature mortality (see Table 10.2). These chronic diseases include type 2 diabetes, hypertension, cardiovascular disease, stroke, breast cancer, endometrial cancer, esophageal cancer, pancreatic cancer, colorectal cancer, chronic pancreatitis, and premature mortality. As shown in Table 10.2, dietary fiber intake reduced the risk of type 2 diabetes by 25%. For women, dietary fiber reduced endometrial cancer risk by 30% and breast cancer risk by 12%. Regardless of gender, dietary fiber reduced the risk of esophageal cancer, stomach cancer, and colorectal cancer by 48%, 46%, and 24%, respectively. For chronic kidney disease patients, dietary fiber intake decreased serum uric acid and serum creatinine levels and mitigated the condition of the disease. In addition, dietary fiber intake reduced the risk of cardiovascular disease mortality, coronary heart disease mortality and cancer mortality by 23%, 24%, and 14%, respectively.

In conclusion, intake of dietary fibers from legumes, whole grains, fruits, and vegetables can lower blood pressure, reduce the risk of type 2 diabetes, cardiovascular disease, and stroke, and the risk of many cancers, including esophageal cancer, stomach cancer, pancreatic cancer, breast cancer, and endometrial cancer. The results support the notion that dietary fibers are excellent food remedies to prevent and treat chronic diseases and cancers.

Table 10.2.   Meta-analytical Confirmation of Dietary Fiber Intake Associated with Lower Risk of Chronic Diseases and Premature Mortality

Chronic Diseases	Reduced Risk, Dietary Fiber
Breast cancer	Dietary fiber intake reduced the risk of breast cancer by 12%. Daily intake of 10 g of dietary fiber reduced the risk of breast cancer by 4%.
Cardiovascular disease	Daily intake of 7 g of dietary fiber reduced the risk of cardiovascular disease by 9% and the risk of coronary heart disease by 9%.
Chronic kidney disease	Foods rich in dietary fiber decreased serum uric acid by 1.76 mmol/L and serum creatinine by 0.42 mg/dL.
Colorectal cancer	Foods rich in dietary fiber reduced the risk of colorectal cancer by 28%. Each additional intake of 10 g of dietary fiber per day reduced the risk of colorectal cancer by 9%.
Endometrial cancer	Foods rich in dietary fiber reduced the risk of endometrial cancer by 30%. Daily intake of 5 g of dietary fiber reduced the risk of endometrial cancer by 18% in women on daily 1,000-calorie diet.

Table 10.2. (*Continued*)

Chronic Diseases	Reduced Risk, Dietary Fiber
Esophageal cancer	Foods rich in dietary fiber reduced the risk of esophageal cancer by 48%. Each additional intake of 10 g of dietary fiber reduced the risk of Barrett's esophagus and esophageal cancer by 31%.
Hypertension	Foods rich in dietary fiber decreased systolic pressure by 0.9 mmHg and diastolic pressure by 0.7 mmHg.
Pancreatic cancer	Foods rich in dietary fiber reduced the risk of pancreatic cancer by 48%. Each additional intake of 10 g of dietary fiber per day reduced the risk of pancreatic cancer by 12%.
Premature mortality	Foods rich in dietary fiber reduced the risk of all-cause mortality, cardiovascular disease mortality, coronary heart disease mortality, and cancer mortality by 16%, 23%, 24%, and 14%, respectively. Daily intake of 10 g of dietary fiber reduced the risk of cardio-vascular disease mortality, coronary heart disease mortality, and cancer mortality by 9%, 11%, and 6%, respectively.
Stomach cancer	Foods rich in dietary fiber reduced the risk of stomach cancer by 42%. Daily intake of 10 g of dietary fiber reduced the risk of stomach cancer by 44%.
Stroke	Foods rich in dietary fiber reduced the risk of stroke by 13%. Daily intake of 10 g of dietary fiber reduced the risk of stroke by 12%.
Type 2 diabetes	Foods rich in dietary fiber decreased fasting glucose level by 9.97 mg/dL and HbA1c by 0.55%. Dietary fibers from whole grains, fruits and vegetables reduced the risk of type 2 diabetes by 25%, 5%, and 7%, respectively. Dietary fiber supplement decreased fasting glucose level by 15.5 mg/dL and HbA1C by 0.26%.

• Recommendation

Prevention — For people at risk of chronic disease: the recommended amount of dietary fiber for men is ½ cup cooked legumes twice per week, and the recommended amount of dietary fiber for women is ⅓ cup of cooked legumes twice per week.

Treatment — For chronic patients: the recommended amount of dietary fiber for men is ½ cup of cooked legumes three times per week, and the recommended amount of dietary fiber for women is ⅓ cup of cooked legumes three times per week.

Materials: Legumes, such as lentils, lima beans, and peas, are the best food sources of dietary fiber. One cup of cooked lentils is about 172 g, which contains 16 g of dietary fiber.

11

Fish

How are fish classified?

Fish can be divided into three major types: jawless fish, cartilage fish, and bony fish. Seven-gill eel and blind eel are jawless fish, and shark and stingray are cartilage fish. Most of the fish humans eat are bony fish, including codfish, sardine, flounder, grouper, anchovy, trout, mackerel, catfish, tuna, and swordfish.

Fish has been an important part of human diet since the hunter-gathering era. Isotope studies provided evidence that fresh-water fish was a major staple for Beijing Tian-Yuan people about 40,000 years ago. From fish drawings on pre-historical cave walls or ancient Egyptian tomb murals, historians concluded that fish was an important part of diets for early human beings. Ancient civilizations of the world, including China, Greece, Roman, Japan, and Europe, all had detailed records on how their ancestors harvested and farmed fish, and how important fish was to the development of their respective cultures. For example, in the 7th to10th centuries, the Chinese people in the Tang Dynasty were fond of having carps as pet fish. The word "carp" in Chinese language sounded like "Lee", and Lee during that era was the last name of the Emperor of the Tang Dynasty. The Emperor felt insulted that people dared to play with "Lee" fish and ordered to ban carps as pet fish. Thereafter, for a rather long period of time, no carp fish could be found in China. In another instance, from the 14th to 16th centuries, the Japanese wrapped fresh fish meat with the rice. This Japanese cuisine is called sushi and is now one of most recognized and loved seafood delicacies in the world.

The following is a brief history of five common types of seafood.

Lobster — Lobsters live on the continental shelf of the Pacific Ocean, Atlantic Ocean, and Indian Ocean. Wild lobsters can live up to 45 to 50 years old. While the reproductive prowess of humans decreases with age, lobsters remain reproductively active at old ages. Scientists believe that the lobster's longevity is probably due to its high level of telomerase, an enzyme that lengthens telomeres at the end of chromosomes. Longer telomeres in chromosomes correlate to longer lifespan in animals, including humans. High telomerase enzyme content may also allow lobsters to repair and grow missing limbs. In the 18th century, dead lobsters were piled up as high as 2 feet tall along the seashore of Boston, Massachusetts. The Bostonians did not like eating lobsters, but they cooked them to feed their workers. Lobster became a poor man's food. To protect the workers, the Massachusetts government declared that feeding workers with lobster meal was an abusive act, and it enacted a law stipulating that any employer could not feed lobster meals to his workers more than 3 times per week. Today, lobster is considered expensive seafood. It may cost you dearly if you like to enjoy three lobster meals in a week.

Salmon — About 20,000 years ago during the Ice Age, a band of people from Central Asia walked across the frozen Bering Sea and reached Alaska. These first Americans soon found large quantities of salmon in the rivers and streams of this new land. Salmon became a part of the native American diet as well as a part of culinary cultures of these people who intended to live in harmony with the nature. For the following thousands of years, the salmon population and its ecosystem remained unchanged in Alaska. However, in the 17th to 19th centuries, new European immigrants built dams and caught huge quantities of salmon annually, which resulted in the destruction of the salmon population and its ecosystem in both the East and West Coasts of the country. To protect salmon population and its ecosystem, the United States Congress enacted a law in 1921 that limits annual salmon catches and allows 50% of Alaskan salmon to return to their spawning streams. That law and its stipulations have effectively protected Alaskan salmon population and its ecosystem to this day.

Mackerel — Mackerel is a major source of seafood around the world. In 2009, five million tons of wild mackerel were caught globally. Almost every ocean in the world produces mackerel. Mackerel has a torpedo-like body shape with beautiful colors, and can grow to a length of 30 to 60 cm and live in groups. Like salmon, mackerel meat is rich in omega-3 fatty acids. Once caught, mackerel spoils easily if it is not immediately frozen. Because of that, salted mackerel or smoked mackerel products are commonly available in the grocery stores in the United States. The mercury content of mackerel varies depending on its ocean environments. Mackerels living in the South Atlantic Ocean have higher mercury contents compared to those living in the North Atlantic Ocean and the Pacific Ocean. Norway catches wild mackerels but also manages farmed mackerels along its coastal regions. The government of Norway strictly limits annual commercial mackerel catches to maintain sustainable mackerel population and its ecosystems. South Norway region named mackerel as its state fish.

Tuna — Tuna is a collective term of several different types of fish. The Pacific Ocean alone has four different types of tuna: bonito fish, yellowfin tuna, bigeye tuna, and longfin tuna. Americans love tuna and consume it either fresh or in cans; tuna sandwiches are a favorite American food. Canned tuna is often made from bonito fish or longfin tuna. Overfishing due to high demand of tuna puts dire pressure on the wild tuna population. Recently, environmental activists and organizations have increased efforts concerning ocean sustainability and indigenous inhabitants, which has led the gradual return of wild tuna population. It is worth noting that blue fin tuna is still listed as an endangered species.

Swordfish — Swordfish are big ocean fish, averaging 5 to 8 feet long and 150 to 250 pounds in weight. The upper jaw of swordfish evolved to become a long and flat like a sword, which is why it is called swordfish. Swordfish lives in the Pacific Ocean, Atlantic Ocean, and Indian Ocean and can swim at a great speed and distance — in less than 21 days, a swordfish can swim from one major ocean to the other. To cope with cold temperature in the deep sea, swordfish are equipped with brain heaters that can raise the temperature in the brain and eyes and increase blood circulation in those regions when it dives into cold deep-sea environments. Fewer than 20 different types of fishes in the world are equipped with brain heaters. Swordfish steak can be found in the menu of seafood restaurants around the world. Owing to its high mercury content, it is recommended not to eat swordfish steak more than once per week. Pregnant women should eschew eating any swordfish meat.

What are the major nutrients in fish?

Fish is an integral part of a healthy diet. Fish contains high levels of polyunsaturated fatty acids, such as omega-3 fatty acids, and are also rich in vitamins and essential elements, including iron, zinc, calcium, Vitamin A, Vitamin B1, Vitamin B6, and Vitamin D. Fish consumption can protect the cardiovascular system and enhance the growth and development of the brain, particularly in children. Table 11.1 depicts the major nutrient contents of twenty different kinds of seafood. It is worth pointing out that mackerel, salmon, and white fish are excellent sources of omega-3 fatty acids, and lobster, shrimp, and squid contain the highest amounts of cholesterol. In addition, shellfish such as blue crab, lobster, oyster, shrimp, and squid contain alarmingly high levels of sodium.

Table 11.1. The Major Nutrients in Common Seafood

Seafood, Cooked (3 ounces)	Total Calorie	Protein (g)	Total Fat (g)	Saturated Fat (g)	Omega-3 Fatty Acid, (mg)	Cholesterol (mg)	Sodium (mg)
Blue crab	90	19	1	0	400	80	310
Catfish	120	19	5	1	300	60	65
Oyster (small, 12)	130	22	2	0	200	60	95
Codfish	90	19	1	0	100	50	60
Flounder	100	20	1	0	400	50	85
Sablefish	90	20	1	0	200	60	70
Lobster	100	20	1	0	100	100	320
Mackerel	190	21	12	3	1,000	60	95
Oyster (mid-size, 12)	120	12	4	1	700	90	190
Trout	130	22	4	1	600	60	30
Grouper	100	20	2	0	400	40	65
Salmon (Atlantic)	150	22	7	1	1,600	50	50
Scallop (large, 6)	150	29	1	0	200	40	70
Striped bass	100	20	2	1	600	40	70
Shrimp	110	22	2	0	300	160	155
Shark	140	22	5	1	NA	50	85
Squid	150	15	6	2	500	220	260
Swordfish	130	21	4	1	700	40	110
Tuna	120	25	1	0	200	50	40
Whitefish	140	20	6	1	1,400	60	55

The data adapted from the 1987 USDA sources.

What Types of Chronic Disease can be Prevented by Consuming Fish?

• Meta-analysis

Cardiovascular disease — Frequent consumption of fish reduces the risk of cardiovascular disease.

A meta-analysis of 26 prospective studies and 12 double-blind randomized clinical trials investigated the relationship between fish intake and cardiovascular disease in 794,000 people including 34,817 cardiovascular disease patients. The results showed that consumption of 2 to 4 servings of fish per week reduced the risk of cerebrovascular disease by 6%, while consumption of more than 5 servings of fish per week reduced the risk of cerebrovascular disease by 12%. Further analysis revealed that the wide range of nutrients in fish, other than omega-3 fatty acids, might have beneficial effects on cerebrovascular health.

Cognitive impairment — Frequent consumption of fish and/or omega-3 fatty acids reduces the risk of cognitive impairment as well as the risk of dementia and Alzheimer's disease.

Cognitive impairment is a neurological disorder causing notice-able decline in one's cognitive abilities, including memory and executive skills. People with cognitive impairment are at risk of developing dementia and Alzheimer's disease. Twenty-one pro-spective cohort studies evaluated the association between fish intake and cognitive impairment in 181,580 people including 4,438 cognitive impairment and dementia cases. The results showed that consumption of each additional serving of fish per week reduced the risk of cognitive impairment by 5% and the risk of Alzheimer's disease by 7%. In addition, each additional intake of 8 g of polyunsaturated fatty acids per day reduced the risk of cognitive impairment by 29%. Furthermore, each additional intake of 0.1 g of docosahexaenoic acid (DHA) per day reduced the risk of dementia by 14% and the risk of Alzheimer's disease by 37%.

Colorectal cancer — People who regularly consume fish have lower risk of colorectal cancer.

A meta-analysis of 27 prospective studies explored the association between fish consumption and colorectal cancer in 2,325,040 people including 24,115 colorectal cancer cases. The results found that fish consumption reduced the risk of colorectal cancer by 7%.

Dementia — Elderly people who regularly consume fish have lower risk of dementia.

A meta-analysis of nine prospective studies investigated the relationship between fish intake and dementia in 28,754 people reported that fish consumption reduced the risk of dementia by 20%. The dose-response analysis revealed that intake of each additional 100 g of fish per week reduced the risk of dementia by 12%.

Esophageal cancer — Frequent consumption of fish lowers the risk of esophageal cancer.

Twenty-seven research papers studied the association between fish intake and esophageal cancer in 2,325,040 subjects including 24,115 gastrointestinal cancer cases. The results revealed that fish consumption reduced the risk of esophageal cancer by 9%.

Heart disease — Regular consumption of fish brings down the incidence of heart disease.

A meta-analysis of five prospective studies investigated the relationship between fish consumption and heart disease in 170,231 people found that consuming fish once per week, two to four times per week and more than five times per week decreased the risk of heart failure by 9%, 13% and 14%, respectively. A dose-response analysis revealed that consuming each additional 20 g of fish per week reduced the risk of heart failure by 6%.

Liver cancer — People who consume fish regularly have lower risk of liver cancer.

A meta-analysis of 27 prospective studies explored the relationship between fish intake and liver cancer in 2,325,040 people including 24,115 liver cancer cases found that fish intake reduced the risk of liver cancer by 29%.

Lung cancer — Regular consumption of fish curtails the risk of lung cancer.

Twenty research papers evaluated the association between fish consumption and lung cancer including 8,799 lung cancer cases and 17,072 healthy controls revealed that fish consumption reduced the risk of lung cancer by 21%.

Premature mortality — People who regularly consume fish have lower risk of premature death from coronary heart disease.

A meta-analysis of 12 prospective studies investigated the relationship between fish consumption and premature mortality in 627,389 subjects including 57,641 mortality cases showed that fish consumption reduced the risk of all-cause mortality by 6%, and daily intake of 60 g of fish reduced the risk of all-cause mortality by 12%. In short, daily consumption of fish could lower the risk of premature mortality. Another meta-analysis of 17 prospective studies explored the association between fish intake and premature mortality in 315,812 people showed that each additional intake of 15 g of fish per day reduced the risk of coronary heart disease mortality by 6%.

Stroke — Consumption of fish once per week can lower the incidence of stroke.

Nineteen prospective studies explored the association between fish consumption and stroke in 402,127 participants including 10,568 stroke cases found that consumption of one to three servings of fish per month reduced the risk of stroke by 3%, and consumption of one serving of fish per week reduced the risk of stroke by 14%. In addition, consumption of two to four servings of fish per week reduced the risk of stroke by 9%, and consumption of 5 servings of fish per week reduced the risk of stroke by 13%.

• Conclusion

The meta-analytical results as shown in Table 11.2 showed that fish intake lowered the risk of cardiovascular disease, stroke, heart disease, esophageal cancer, lung cancer, liver cancer, colorectal cancer, cognitive impairment, and premature mortality. Specifically, fish

Table 11.2: Meta-analytical Confirmation of Fish Consumption Associated with Lower Risks of Chronic Diseases and Cancers

Chronic Diseases	Reduced Risk, Fish Consumption
Cardiovascular disease	2–4 servings and more than 5 servings of fish per week reduced the risk of cardiovascular disease by 6% and 12%, respectively.
Cognitive impairment	Each additional serving of fish per week reduced the risk of cognitive impairment by 5% and the risk of Alzheimer's disease by 7%. Daily intake of 8 g of polyunsaturated fatty acids reduced the risk of cognitive impairment by 29% and the risk of Parkinson's disease by 10%.
Colorectal cancer	Fish consumption reduced the risk of colorectal cancer by 7%.
Dementia	Fish consumption reduced the risk of dementia by 20%. Weekly intake of 100 g of fish reduced the risk of dementia by 12%. Daily intake of 0.1 g of DHA reduced the risk of dementia by 37%.
Esophageal cancer	Fish consumption reduced the risk of esophageal cancer by 9%.
Heart disease	Fish intake of 1 serving, 2–4 servings, and more than 5 servings per week reduced the risk of heart disease by 9%, 13%, and 14%, respectively. Weekly intake of 20 g of fish reduced the risk of heart failure by 6%.
Liver cancer	Fish consumption reduced the risk of liver cancer by 29%.
Lung cancer	Fish consumption reduced the risk of lung cancer by 21%.
Premature mortality	Fish consumption reduced the risk of premature mortality by 6%. Daily intake of 60 g of fish reduced the risk of all-cause mortality by 12%. Daily intake of 15 g of fish reduced the risk of coronary heart disease mortality by 6%.
Stroke	Fish intake of once per month, once per week, 2–4 times per week, and more than 5 times per week reduced the risk of stroke by 3%, 14%, 9%, and 13%, respectively.

intake reduced the risk of cardiovascular disease, stroke, and dementia by 12%, 13%, 20%, respectively. In addition, fish consumption reduced the risk of esophageal cancer, lung cancer, liver cancer, and colorectal cancer by 9%, 21%, 29%, and 7%, respectively. Fish intake also reduced the risk of cognitive impairment by 29% in elder people. Moreover, consumption of fish reduced the risk of all-cause mortality by 6% and the risk of coronary heart disease mortality by 6%.

In summary, regular fish intake is associated with lower risks of cardiovascular diseases including coronary heart disease and stroke, and it is also associated with lower cancer risks, including lung cancer and gastrointestinal cancers. Adding fish as a part of a healthy diet may prevent cardiovascular diseases and some cancers and may also contribute to a longer and healthier life.

Should you be concerned about mercury content in seafood?

Every year, volcanic eruptions from the earth's surface and seabed release 2,700 to 6,000 tons of mercury vapors into the air, sea, lakes, livers, and ground. In addition, exhaust gases and smoke from coal-burning factories and houses release another 2,000 to 3,000 tons of mercury vapors into the atmosphere annually. Mercury vapors dissolved in water can be converted to toxic methyl mercury by bacteria living in fresh or saltwater environments. Methyl mercury in the river or ocean can get into the tissues and organs of fish or shrimp via the mouth or gills. When consuming fish, we inevitably ingest the methyl mercury that is present in fish meat. There is an old saying that goes "The big fish eat the little fish, the little fish eat small shrimp, and the shrimp eat sludge". This saying is helpful in demonstrating that the large fish higher in the food chain contain the most mercury, because they absorb the mercury from the smaller fish they consume. Shrimp has low mercury content, while larger fish have higher mercury contents.

As shown in Table 11.3, the mercury contents of most of the seafood are in the range of 0.01–0.3 ppm, which is below upper-intake limit of 1 ppm daily as recommended by the United States

Table 11.3.   Mercury Contents in Common Seafood

Seafood	Mercury Content, Average (ppm)	Mercury Content, Mean (ppm)	Seafood	Mercury Content, Average (ppm)	Mercury Content, Mean (ppm)
Scallop	0.003	ND	Trout	0.071	0.025
Clam	0.009	0.002	Herring	0.078	0.042
Shrimp	0.009	0.001	White fish	0.089	0.067
Oyster	0.012	ND	Lobster	0.093	0.062
Sardine	0.013	0.010	Carp	0.110	0.134
Tilapia	0.013	0.004	Codfish	0.111	0.066
Salmon (canned)	0.014	0.010	Tuna (canned)	0.126	0.077
Sablefish	0.016	0.011	Square head fish	0.144	0.099
Salmon (fresh)	0.022	0.015	Red fish	0.166	0.113
Squid	0.024	0.017	Striped bass	0.167	0.094
Catfish	0.024	0.005	Marlin	0.178	0.180
Alaska Codfish	0.031	0.003	Mackerel (Spain)	0.182	N/A
Mackerel (North Atlantic)	0.05	N/A	Striped bass (Chile)	0.354	0.303
Black cod (Atlantic)	0.055	0.049	Tuna (fresh)	0.358	0.36
Flounder	0.056	0.05	Shark	0.979	0.811
Crab	0.065	0.05	Swordfish	0.995	0.87

The data adapted from the United States FDA sources (1990–2012); ND, not detected: N/A, not available.

FDA. Fish such as shark and swordfish have higher mercury contents (see Table 11.3). However, the upper daily intake limit of 1 ppm does not mean that you will fall ill immediately if you ingested 1 ppm of mercury. The daily upper intake limit recommended by the FDA is often set at a dose that is at least 10 times less than the adverse-effect dosage. In other words, symptoms of mercury toxicity may appear when daily intake of mercury exceeds 10 ppm or higher. Nevertheless, avoid eating any high-mercury fish, such as tuna and swordfish; children and pregnant women should be especially careful to avoid these fish.

• Recommendation

Prevention — For people at risk of chronic disease: men should consume 4 ounces of fish 3 times per week, and women should consume 3 ounces of fish 3 times per week.

Treatment — For chronic patients: men should consume 4 ounces of fish 5 times per week, and women should consume 3 ounces of fish 5 times per weeks.

Materials: Select fish with low mercury content, such as cod, sardine, flounder, grouper, anchovy, trout, mackerel, and catfish. A 3-ounce of cooked fish is about the size of Apple iPhone, and a 4-ounce of cooked fish is about the size of a US bank checkbook.

12

Flaxseed

Flaxseed (also called linseed) comes from the flax plant with five-petal blue (to purple) flowers and reddish-brown color seeds. It can grow up to 47 inches with thin leaves and stems. Common flax (Linum usitatissimum) originated in the Mediterranean region and then spread to France, Belgium, Russia, China, Egypt, and the United States. Cultivation of flax dates back thousands of years. Flax remnants were discovered in ancient dwellings in Switzerland, and in Egyptian's mummies.

Flaxseeds contain a high amount of plant-based omega-3 fatty acids and lignans, both of which exert antioxidant and anti-inflammatory properties, neutralize free radicals, inhibit inflammation, support the vascular system, and reduce the risk of hypertension.

What Types of Chronic Disease can be Prevented by Consuming Flaxseeds?

• Meta-analysis

Hypertension — Regular consumption of flaxseeds and/or flaxseed extract supplement lowers blood pressure in hypertensive patients.

Fifteen double-blind randomized clinical trials investigated the relationship between flaxseed intake and hypertension found that consuming flaxseed extract supplement decreased systolic pressure by 2.9 mmHg and diastolic pressure by 2.4 mmHg in hypertensive patients.

• Conclusion

The meta-analytical results demonstrated that hypertensive patients who consumed flaxseed extract supplement decreased systolic pressure by 2.9 mmHg and diastolic pressure by 2.4 mmHg as shown in Table 12.1. In addition, hypertensive patients who consumed whole flaxseed decreased diastolic pressure by 2 mmHg. The results support the view that both flaxseed extract and whole flaxseeds can lower blood pressure in patients with hypertension. Even though the magnitude of the effect is relatively small, a reduction of systolic pressure by 2 mmHg is equivalent to a 10% diminished risk in stroke mortality and a 7% decreased risk in heart disease mortality. Adding flaxseeds to a nutrient-balanced diet may mitigate the condition of the disease in patients with hypertension.

Table 12.1. **Meta-analytical Confirmation of Flaxseed Intake Associated with Reduced Blood Pressure in Hypertensive Patients**

Chronic Disease	Reduced Risk, Flaxseeds
Hypertension	Flaxseed extract decreased systolic pressure by 2.9 mmHg and diastolic pressure by 2.4 mmHg in hypertensive patients.
	Whole flaxseed decreased diastolic pressure by 2 mmHg in hypertensive patients.

• Recommendation

Prevention — For people at risk of hypertension: the recommended amount for men is one teaspoon of flaxseeds twice each day, and the recommended amount for women is ½ teaspoon of flaxseeds twice each day.

Treatment — For hypertensive patients: the recommended amount for men is one teaspoon of flaxseeds three times each day, and the recommended amount for women is ½ teaspoon of flaxseeds three times each day.

Material: Ground flaxseeds are easier to digest and absorb in the intestines compared to whole flaxseeds. When purchasing, select ground flaxseeds or buy whole flaxseeds and grind them at home; you can grind them the same way you grind your coffee beans. Add ground flaxseeds to breakfast cereals or other meals. One teaspoon of ground flaxseeds is about 7 g.

13

Fruits

How are fruits classified?

Fruits are produced after flowers have faded in flowering plants. Ripe fruits are often sweet and tasty. Humans and other animals enjoy eating ripe fruits. In ancient times, the migrations of humans and other animals helped spread the seeds of flowering plants far and wide. Fruits can be divided into five major types: Drupes (peach and plum), Berries (grape, blueberry and strawberry), Pomes (apple and pear), Hesperia (lemon, orange and tangerine), and Pepos (cantaloupe).

What are the major nutrients in fruits?

Fruits with high water contents are low fat, low sodium, and low-calorie foods. They are excellent food sources of dietary fiber, antioxidant Vitamin A and Vitamin C, and contain no cholesterol. Table 13.1 lists the major nutrients in 21 common fruits. Fruits contain high amounts of potassium but low amounts of sodium. In addition, apples, bananas, and kiwi fruits contain abundant amounts of potassium and dietary fiber. Among 21 different types of fruits shown in Table 13.1, pear has the highest amount of dietary fiber, and cantaloupe has the highest amount of Vitamin A. The best food sources for Vitamin C are cantaloupe, grapefruit, kiwi fruit, and orange. One mid-sized kiwi fruit contains 240 mg of Vitamin C, which fulfills the daily requirement for Vitamin C.

Table 13.1.   The Major Nutrients in Common Fruits

Fruits	Amount, Consumed, g	Sodium, mg	Potassium, mg	Dietary Fiber, g	Vitamin A, %DV	Vitamin C, %DV
Apple	242	0	260	5	2	8
Avocado	30	0	140	1	0	4
Banana	126	0	450	3	2	15
Cantaloupe	134	20	240	1	120	80
Grapefruit	154	0	160	2	35	100
Grape	126	15	240	1	0	2
Melon	134	30	210	1	2	45
Kiwi fruit	148	0	450	4	2	240
Lemon	58	0	75	2	0	40
Lime	67	0	75	2	0	35
Nectarine	140	0	250	2	8	15
Orange	154	0	250	3	2	130
Peach	147	0	230	2	6	15
Pear	166	0	190	6	0	10
Pineapple	112	10	120	1	2	50
Plum	151	0	230	2	8	10
Strawberry	147	0	170	2	0	160
Sweet cherry	140	0	350	1	2	15
Tangerine	109	0	160	2	6	45
Watermelon	280	0	270	1	30	25

Data adapted from the 2008 United States FDA sources; %DV, % daily value, based on daily intake of 2,000 calories.

What Types of Chronic Disease can be Prevented by Consuming Fruits?

• Meta-analysis

Breast cancer — Women who regularly consume fruits have lower risk of breast cancer.

A meta-analysis of 24 prospective studies investigated the relationship between fruit consumption and breast cancer in 15,631 women found that consumption of fruits reduced the risk of breast cancer by 32%.

Colorectal cancer — People who regularly consume fruits have lower risks of colorectal cancer.

Nine clinical trial reports examined the relationship between fruit intake and colorectal cancer including 2,006 colorectal cancer cases and 3,504 control subjects. The results revealed that consumption of fruits reduced the risk of colorectal cancer by 15%.

Endometrial cancer — Women who consume fruits daily have lower risks of endometrial cancer.

Seventeen clinical reports investigated the relationship between fruit consumption and endometrial cancer showed that consuming fruits reduced the risk of endometrial cancer by 10%. In addition, daily consumption of 100 g of fruits reduced the risk of endometrial cancer by 3%.

Esophageal adenocarcinoma — Frequent consumption of fruits lessens the risk of esophageal adenocarcinoma.

Twelve research articles evaluated the association between fruit consumption and esophageal adenocarcinoma including 1,572 esophageal adenocarcinoma cases showed that fruit consumption reduced the risk of esophageal adenocarcinoma by 27%.

Esophageal cancer — People who frequently consume fruits have lower incident rates of esophageal cancer.

Another meta-analysis of 32 clinical trials studied the relationship between fruit consumption and esophageal cancer including 10,037 esophageal cancer cases. The results showed that frequent consumption of fruits reduced the risk of esophageal cancer by 47%.

Hypertension — Regular consumption of fruits brings down the risk of hypertension.

Nine prospective studies explored the association between fruit consumption and hypertension in 185,676 people found that consumption of fruits reduced the risk of hypertension by 13%. The dose-response data revealed that each additional serving of fruits per day decreased the risk of hypertension by 1.9%.

Lung cancer — Daily consumption of fruits curtails the risk of lung cancer.

A meta-analysis of 72 prospective studies examined the relationship between fruit consumption and lung cancer in 36,678 people found that consumption of fruits reduced the risk of lung cancer by 18%. Quantitative studies revealed that each additional intake of 100 g of fruits per day reduced the risk of lung cancer by 8%.

Oral cancer — People who consume fruits daily greatly lower the risk of oral cancer.

Sixteen research articles evaluated the association between fruit consumption and oral cancer reported that each additional serving of fruits per day reduced the risk of oral cancer by 49%.

Pancreatic cancer — Regular fruit consumption can cut down the risk of pancreatic cancer.

A meta-analysis of eleven prospective studies evaluated the relationship between fruit consumption and pancreatic cancer found that consumption of fruits reduced the risk of pancreatic cancer by 29%.

Premature mortality — People who consume fruits daily have lower risks of premature mortality and breast cancer survivals who consume fruits regularly can trim down the risk of premature death from breast cancer.

A meta-analysis of 16 prospective studies investigated the relationship between fruit intake and premature mortality in 833,234 people including 28,329 mortality cases. The results showed that each additional serving of fruits daily reduced the risk of all-cause mortality by 6%. Another meta-analysis of 10 prospective studies examined the association between fruit consumption and premature mortality including 31,210 breast cancer mortality cases revealed that consumption of fruits reduced the risk of breast cancer mortality by 13%.

Stroke — Daily fruit consumption can significantly lower the risk of stroke.

A meta-analysis of 12 prospective studies explored the relationship between fruit intake and stroke in 760,629 subjects including 16,981 stroke cases found that each additional daily intake of 200 g of fruits reduced the risk of stroke by 32%.

Type 2 diabetes — Daily consumption of fruits curtails the risk of type 2 diabetes.

Nine prospective studies examined the association between fruit consumption and type 2 diabetes in 403,259 people including 27,940 type 2 diabetes cases revealed that daily consumption of 200 g of fruits reduced the risk of type 2 diabetes by 13%.

• Conclusion

The meta-analytical data presented in Table 13.2 showed that consumption of fruits reduced the risk of ten chronic diseases and premature mortality. These ten chronic diseases include hypertension, type 2 diabetes, stroke, oral cancer, esophageal cancer, lung cancer, breast cancer, endometrial cancer, pancreatic cancer, and colorectal cancer. Specifically, consumption of fruits reduced the risk of stroke, hypertension, and type 2 diabetes by 32%, 13%, and 13%, respectively. In addition, consumption of fruits reduced the risk of gastrointestinal cancers, including oral cancer, esophageal cancer, pancreatic cancer, and colorectal cancer by 49%, 47%, 29%, and 15%, respectively. Moreover, consumption of fruits reduced the risk of lung cancer by 18%. Women who consumed fruits lowered the risk of breast cancer by 32% and the risk of endometrial cancer by 10%. Furthermore, consumption of fruits reduced the risk of all-cause mortality by 8% and the risk of breast cancer mortality by 13%.

In summary, fruit intake can lower the risk of hypertension, stroke and type 2 diabetes and the risk of lung cancer, gastrointestinal cancers including oral cancer, esophageal cancer, pancreatic cancer, and colorectal cancer, and gynecological cancers including breast cancer and endometrial cancer, and premature mortality. Adding fruits to a healthy balanced diet may prevent chronic disease as well as increase lifespan.

Table 13.2. Meta-analytical Confirmation of Fruit Consumption Associated with Lower Risks of Chronic Diseases

Chronic Diseases	Reduced Risk, Fruit Consumption
Breast cancer	Fruits reduced the risk of breast cancer by 32%.
Colorectal cancer	Fruits reduced the risk of colorectal cancer by 15%.
Endometrial cancer	Fruit reduced the risk of endometrial cancer by 10%. Daily intake of 100 g of fruits reduced the risk of endometrial cancer by 3%.
Esophageal adenocarcinoma	Fruits reduced the risk of esophageal adenocarcinoma by 27%.
Esophageal cancer	Fruits reduced the risk of esophageal cancer by 47%.
Hypertension	Fruits reduced the risk of hypertension by 13%. Each additional serving of fruits per day reduced the risk of hypertension by 1.9%.
Lung cancer	Fruits reduced the risk of lung cancer by 18%. Each additional intake of 100 g of fruits per day reduced the risk of lung cancer by 8%.
Oral cancer	Fruits reduced the risk of oral cancer by 49%.
Pancreatic cancer	Fruits reduced the risk of pancreatic cancer by 29%.
Premature mortality	Fruits reduced the risk of all-cause mortality and breast cancer mortality by 6% and 13%, respectively.
Stroke	Daily intake of 200 g of fruits reduced the risk of stroke by 32%.
Type 2 diabetes	Daily intake of 200 g of fruits reduced the risk of type 2 diabetes by 13%.

• Recommendation

Prevention — For people at risk of chronic diseases: men should consume ½ cup of chopped fresh fruits, three times per day, and women should consume ½ cup of chopped fresh fruits, twice per day.

Treatment — For chronic disease patients: men should consume one cup of chopped fresh fruits, twice per day, and women should consume ½ cup of chopped fresh fruits, three times per day.

Materials: Daily, choose five different types of fruits, including apple and orange. One cup of chopped fresh fruits is about 175 grams.

14

Garlic

Garlic belongs to the allium family of vegetables, which also include onions, scallions, and leeks. Garlic originated in Central Asia and has been one of the oldest known food flavoring and seasoning plant worldwide. Human consumption of garlic dates back at least five thousand years. Historical records have shown that garlic was domesticated in Central Asia around 3000 BCE and spread to the Mediterranean region and Europe. Garlic cloves were found in the tomb of the famous pharaoh Tutankhamen in Egypt. Besides being used as a seasoning, since ancient times, garlic has been used to prevent and treat a variety of illness, from abdominal pain to fever, hypertension, diabetes, infections, arthritis, and the like.

Garlic contains a high amount of organic sulfur compounds, of which the most well-known is allicin. The pungent smell of garlic is due to organic sulfur compounds. These organic sulfur compounds including allicin, through their antioxidant activities, contribute protection against free radical damage in the body. In addition to organic sulfur compounds, garlic also contains flavonoids, manganese, selenium, copper, Vitamin B1, and Vitamin B6.

What Types of Chronic Disease can be Prevented by Consuming Garlic?

• Meta-analysis

Hypercholesterolemia — Garlic powder intake can favorably lower blood cholesterol levels in hypercholesterolemic patients.

Fifty-seven double-blind randomized clinical trials investigated the relationship between garlic consumption and hypercholesterolemia found that consumption of garlic powder decreased total cholesterol by 15.4 mg/dL and LDL cholesterol by 8.1 mg/dL in patients with hypercholesterolemia.

Hypertension — Garlic consumption can lower blood pressure in both pre-hypertensive individuals and hypertensive patients.

Twenty double-blind randomized clinical trials explored the association between garlic consumption and hypertension reported that garlic consumption decreased systolic pressure by 5.1 mmHg and diastolic pressure by 2.5 mmHg in pre-hypertensive patients. In hypertensive patients, garlic decreased systolic pressure by 8.7 mmHg and diastolic pressure by 6.1 mmHg.

Prostate cancer — Garlic intake curtails the risk of prostate cancer.

Six research papers examined the relationship between garlic intake and prostate cancer found that garlic consumption reduced the risk of prostate cancer by 23%.

Stomach cancer — People who consume garlic daily have lower risk of stomach cancer.

A meta-analysis of twenty-one research articles investigated the relationship between garlic consumption and stomach cancer in 542,220 people revealed that habitual intake of allium garlic reduced the risk of stomach cancer by 40%, and each additional intake of 20 g of garlic per day reduced the risk of stomach cancer by 9%.

Type 2 diabetes — Regular consumption of garlic and/or garlic powder lowers fasting glucose levels in pre-diabetic individuals and type 2 diabetic patients, as well as reduces the risk of type 2 diabetes in pre-diabetic individuals and improves the condition of the disease in type 2 diabetic patients.

Four double-blind randomized clinical trials evaluated the relationship between garlic powder intake and type 2 diabetes showed that intake of garlic powder decreased the fasting glucose level by 17.3 mg/dL in type 2 diabetic patients. Analysis confirms that garlic powder intake lessens the risk of type 2 diabetes. Additional supporting evidence about the benefits of garlic is documented in a meta-analysis, which revealed that garlic consumption deceased the fasting glucose level by 1.7 mg/dL in pre-diabetic individuals.

• Conclusion

As confirmed by the meta-analytical data in Table 14.1, garlic consumption reduced the risk of hypertension, hypercholesterolemia,

Table 14.1. Meta-analytic Confirmation of Garlic Intake Associated with Lower Risks of 5 Chronic Diseases

Chronic Disease	Risk Reduction, Garlic
Hypercholesterolemia	Garlic decreased total cholesterol level by 15.4 mg/dL and LDL cholesterol level by 8.1 mg/dL in patients with hypercholesterolemia.
Hypertension	Pre-hypertensive individuals who regularly consumed garlic decreased systolic pressure by 5.1 mmHg and diastolic pressure by 2.5 mmHg. Hypertensive patients who regularly consumed garlic decreased systolic pressure by 8.7 mmHg and diastolic pressure by 6.1 mmHg.
Prostate cancer	Garlic reduced the risk of prostate cancer by 23%.
Stomach cancer	Garlic reduced the risk of stomach cancer by 40%. Daily intake of 20 g of garlic reduced the risk of stomach cancer by 9%.
Type 2 diabetes	Diabetic patients who regularly consumed garlic decreased fasting blood glucose level by 17.3 mg/dL. Pre-diabetic individuals who regularly consumed garlic decreased fasting blood glucose level by 1.7 mg/dL.

type 2 diabetes, stomach cancer, and prostate cancer. Hypertensive patients who regularly consumed garlic decreased systolic pressure by 8.7 mmHg and diastolic pressure by 6.1 mmHg, and pre-hypertensive individuals who regularly consumed garlic decreased systolic pressure by 5.1 mmHg and diastolic pressure by 2.5 mmHg. Garlic is also shown to decrease the total cholesterol level by 8.1 mg/dL and LDL cholesterol level by 15.4 mg/dL in patients with hypercholesterolemia. In addition, type 2 diabetic patients who consumed garlic reduced their fasting blood glucose level by 17.3 mg/dL, and pre-type 2 diabetic patients who consumed garlic reduced their fasting blood glucose level by 1.7 mg/dL. Furthermore, consuming garlic reduced the risk of stomach cancer by 46% and the risk of prostate cancer by 23%.

The results are consistent with the view that garlic intake can lower blood pressure in hypertensive patients, improve blood cholesterol profiles in hypercholesterolemic patients, reduce the fasting blood glucose level in both type 2 diabetic patients and pre-diabetic individuals, and decrease the risk of stomach cancer and prostate cancer. It is recommended that garlic be included in a healthy diet to prevent chronic diseases and cancers.

• Recommendation

Prevention — For people at risk of chronic disease: men should consume 1 teaspoon of chopped raw garlic, twice daily or ¼ teaspoon of garlic powder supplement, twice daily, and women should consume ½ teaspoon of chopped raw garlic, twice daily or ¼ teaspoon of garlic powder supplement, twice daily.

Treatment — For chronic disease patients: men should consume 1 teaspoon of chopped raw garlic, three times daily or ½ teaspoon of garlic powder supplement, three times daily, and women should consume one teaspoon of chopped raw garlic, three times daily or ¼ teaspoon of garlic powder supplement, three times daily.

Material: Raw garlic contains allicin, which is lost once cooked. Only raw garlic exerts medicinal effects. Chopped raw garlic may be added directly to cooked meals. Allicin contents in garlic powder supplements vary greatly. Select the supplement product which contains at least 150 mg of allicin in one gram of garlic powder. Again, garlic powder can be added directly to cooked meals.

15

Ginger

Ginger is a native plant of Southeast Asia and its use in China and India dates back thousands of years. By the 1st century, explorers had taken ginger to the Mediterranean region. The Greeks and Romans used ginger for its culinary and medicinal purposes. By the 11th century, ginger was a well-known spice in England and soon it spread to the rest of Europe.

Since ancient times, ginger has been used for treating a myriad of human illness, such as cataract, rheumatoid arthritis, asthma, stroke, constipation, type 2 diabetes, and etcetera. Gingers are rich in phenolic compounds, including curcumin and shogaol, both of which exhibit antioxidant activities by inhibiting oxidative damage and preventing atherosclerosis. In addition, curcumin and shogaol exert anti-inflammatory activities in inhibiting the production of inflammatory mediators, including leukotrienes, prostaglandins, tumor necrosis factors and interferon-1. Ginger can also stimulate the liver to produce bile acid, accelerate the excretion of cholesterol and bile juice from the gallbladder, and lower blood cholesterol level.

What Types of Chronic Disease can be Prevented by Consuming Ginger?

• Meta-analysis

Hypercholesterolemia — Regular consumption of ginger lowers blood cholesterol level and improves blood lipid profiles in hypercholesterolemic patients.

A meta-analysis of nine prospective studies investigated the relationship between ginger consumption and hypercholesterolemia found that ginger consumption increased the HDL cholesterol level by 1.2 mg/dL and decreased triglycerides by 1.6 mg/dL in patients with hypercholesterolemia.

• Conclusion

Table 15.1 shows that regular consumption of ginger increased the HDL cholesterol level by 1.2 mg/dL and decreased triglycerides by 1.6 mg/dL in patients with high blood cholesterol levels. The results confirm that ginger is effective in lowering blood cholesterol levels and improving blood lipid profiles in patients with hypercholesterolemia. Including ginger to a nutrient-balanced diet can lower blood cholesterol levels and may improve the condition of the disease in patients with hypercholesterolemia.

Table 15.1. Meta-analytical Confirmation of Ginger Consumption Associated with Improved Blood Lipid Profiles in Patients with Hypercholesterolemia

Chronic Disease	Reduced Risk, Ginger Intake
Hypercholesterolemia	Hypercholesterolemic patients who regularly consumed ginger decreased triglycerides by 1.6 mg/dL and increased HDL cholesterol level by 1.2 mg/dL.

• Recommendation

Prevention — For people at risk of hypercholesterolemia: the recommended dose for men is one teaspoon of raw ginger powder twice per day, and the recommended dose for women is ½ teaspoon of raw ginger powder twice per day.

Treatment — For hypercholesterolemic patients: the recommended dose for men is one teaspoon of raw ginger powder three times per day, and the recommended dose for women is ½ teaspoon of raw ginger powder three times per day.

Material: Select fresh organic ginger, peer the skin, grind it to powder and mix it with your favorite cooked meals. One teaspoon of raw ginger powder is about 1.8 g.

16

Grape Seed Extract

Among all fruits, which fruit has the largest production in the world? Many people guess bananas, oranges, or apples. In fact, the answer is grapes. Each year more than 72 million tons of grapes are produced in the world. The history of grape cultivation is parallel to the history of humankind. Archeological evidence revealed that in the Paleolithic Era, humans domesticated the grape plant. In 4000 BCE, grapes and wines were abundant in the Mediterranean region. Grape cultivation and winery techniques subsequently spread from the Mediterranean region to Italy, Spain, and France, countries that have had a long history of wine culture. In the mid-20th century, the West Coast of the United States, particularly Northern California, emerged as a new region for the high-quality wine production in the world. Globally, less than 12% grapes produced are consumed as fresh grapes and the rest are earmarked for wine producing purposes.

Grape seed extract is rich in polyphenols, such as proanthocyanidins. Proanthocyanidins exhibit strong antioxidant properties by neutralizing free radicals, preventing free radical-induced oxidative damage, and protecting the heart and vascular system. French diets are generally high in saturated fats, such as butter, but the French people seem to have a lower incident rate of cardiovascular diseases compared to the Americans. This contradictory phenomenon was dubbed "French paradox". This paradoxical observation is in part attributed to the French's consumption of heart healthy red wines. Like grape seed extract, red wines also contain abundant amounts of antioxidant polyphenols. Grapes, dark chocolate, flaxseeds, clove, and chestnuts are all excellent food sources of polyphenols.

What Types of Chronic Disease can be Prevented by Consuming Grape Seed Extract?

• Meta-analysis

Hypertension — Grape seed extract intake can favorably lower blood pressure in hypertensive patients with various health conditions.

Sixteen double-blind randomized clinical trials explored the relationship between grape seed extract intake and hypertension found that in hypertensive patients, grape seed extract decreased systolic pressure by 6.1 mmHg and diastolic pressure by 2.8 mmHg. In middle-aged hypertensive patients, grape seed extract decreased systolic pressure by 6.0 mmHg and diastolic pressure by 3.1 mmHg. In obese hypertensive patients, grape seed extract decreased systolic pressure by 4.5 mmHg. In addition, in hypertensive patients with metabolic syndrome, grape seed extract decreased systolic pressure by 8.5 mmHg.

• Conclusion

In patients with hypertension, grape seed extract decreased systolic pressure by 6.1 mmHg and diastolic pressure by 2.8 mmHg in hypertensive patients (see Table 16.1). Additionally, in obese hypertensive patients, grape seed extract decreased systolic pressure by 4.5 mmHg, and in hypertensive patients with metabolic syndromes, grape seed extract decreased systolic pressure by 8.5 mmHg. Therefore, grape seed extract can noticeably lower blood pressure of hypertensive patients, regardless of their ages and other health conditions. The results provide strong evidence that grape seed extract is an efficacious food remedy to prevent and treat hypertension.

Table 16.1.　Meta-analytical Confirmation of Grape Seed Extract Associated with Reduced Blood Pressure in Patients with Hypertension

Chronic Disease	Reduced Risk, Grape Seed Extract
Hypertension	Hypertensive patients who regularly consumed grape seed extract decreased systolic pressure by 6.1 mmHg and diastolic pressure by 2.8 mmHg. Middle-aged hypertensive patients who regularly consumed grape seed extract decreased systolic pressure by 6.0 mmHg and diastolic pressure by 3.1 mmHg. Obese hypertensive patients who regularly consumed grape seed extract decreased systolic pressure by 4.5 mmHg. Hypertensive patients who metabolic syndrome who regularly consumed grape seed extract decreased systolic pressure by 8.5 mmHg.

• Recommendation

Prevention — For people at risk of hypertension: the recommended dose for men is 200 mg of grape seed extract daily, and the recommended dose for women is 100 mg of grape seed extract daily.

Treatment — For hypertensive patients: the recommended dose for men is 500 mg of grape seed extract daily, and the recommended dose for women is 300 mg of grape seed extract daily.

Material: Polyphenols, such as proanthocyanidins, are active ingredients in grape seed extract. Select grape seed extract supplements that contain at least 80% polyphenols.

17

Legumes

Legumes are the third largest flowering plants on Earth, with more than 20,000 different species. They can grow in a great variety of ecosystems, from mountains to plains to deserts. Legumes were among the first cultivated plants in the Mediterranean region. Chickpea, lentils, and broad beans are all native plants of the Near Eastern Mediterranean region. Nitrogen-fixation bacteria living in nodules on the roots of legumes can obtain nitrogen from the atmosphere, which goes into the production of proteins. Therefore, legumes have the highest protein contents of all plant foods.

Legumes include chickpeas, broad beans, black beans, red beans, lentils, kidney beans, lima beans, and the like. In addition, legumes contain concentrated amounts of B vitamins, iron, calcium, phosphorous, zinc, and magnesium. They are excellent food sources of antioxidants, folate and dietary fiber.

Hypercholesterolemia and type 2 diabetes are the two major risk factors for obesity. Legume proteins support the syntheses of cholecystokinin and glucagon-like peptides in the digestive tract. Cholecystokinin can stimulate the gallbladder to contract and release bile juices with cholesterol to the intestines and result in reducing blood cholesterol level. Glucagon-like peptides, on the other hand, can support insulin secretion from the pancreas and result in decreasing the blood glucose level. Thus, legume protein intake may lower the risk of hypercholesterolemia, and thereby reduce the risk of obesity.

Moreover, legumes are rich in flavonoids, of which flavonoid fisetin is known to bind and disrupt the microtubule structure of cancerous cells, block the cell cycle, inhibit the growth and tumorigenesis, and reduce the risk of cancers.

What Types of Chronic Disease can be Prevented by Consuming Legumes?

• Meta-analysis

Colorectal cancer — Regular consumption of legumes curtails the risk of colorectal cancer.

Fourteen case-control studies investigated the relationship between legume consumption and colorectal cancer in 1,903,459 participants, of which 12,261 were colorectal cancer cases. The meta-analytical results showed that consumption of legumes reduced the risk of colorectal cancer by 18%.

Colorectal adenomas — People who consume legumes regularly have lower risk of colorectal adenomas.

The meta-analysis of fourteen research papers examined the association between legume consumption and colorectal adenomas in 101,856 people, including 8,380 colorectal cancer cases. The results revealed that consumption of legumes reduced the risk of colorectal adenomas by 17%.

Heart disease — Regular consumption of legumes lessens the risk of heart disease.

A meta-analysis of 25 research papers evaluated the relationship between legume consumption and heart disease in 501,791 participants including 11,869 ischemic heart disease cases. The results showed that consumption of 100 g of legumes 4 times per week decreased the risk of ischemic heart disease by 14%.

Hypercholesterolemia — Legume consumption lowers blood cholesterol levels and improves lipoprotein profiles in patients with hypercholesterolemia.

Ten double-blind randomized clinical trials investigated the association between legume consumption and hypercholesterolemia found that consumption of legumes decreased the total cholesterol level by 11.8 mg/dL and LDL cholesterol level by 8.0 mg/dL in hypercholesterolemic patients.

Obesity — People who regularly consume legumes lose weight and have lower risk of obesity.

Twenty-one double-blind randomized clinical trials examined the relationship between legume consumption and obesity showed that daily consumption of legumes for 4 weeks reduced 0.75 lb in body weight.

Prostate cancer — Elderly people who frequently consume legumes can thwart the risk of prostate cancer.

A meta-analysis of ten research articles evaluated the association between legume consumption and prostate cancer in 281,034 people including 10,234 prostate cancer cases found that consumption of legumes reduced the risk of prostate cancer by 15%. The dose-response studies revealed that each additional intake of 20 g of legumes per day reduced the risk of prostate cancer by 3.5%.

• Conclusion

Table 17.1 shows that consuming legumes reduced the risk of five chronic diseases including obesity, hypercholesterolemia, heart disease, prostate cancer, and colorectal cancer. Specifically, legume consumption reduced weight in overweight and obese individuals by 0.75 lb. In addition, hypercholesterolemic patients who consumed legumes reduced the total cholesterol level by 11.8 mg/dL and LDL cholesterol level by 8.0 mg/dL. Furthermore, legume consumption reduced the risk of ischemic heart disease, prostate cancer, and colorectal cancer by 14%, 15%, and 18%, respectively.

In summary, legume intake can lead to weight loss in overweight and obese individuals, improve the blood lipid prolife in patients with high blood cholesterol, and reduce the risk of heart disease, prostate cancer, and colorectal cancer. Legumes should be included in the dietary recommendations for the prevention and management of obesity, hypercholesterolemia, heart disease, prostate cancer, and colorectal cancer.

Table 17.1. Meta-analytical Confirmation of Legume Consumption Associated with Lower Risk of Chronic Diseases

Chronic Diseases	Reduced Risk, Legumes
Colorectal cancer	Legumes reduced the risk of colorectal cancer by 18%.
	Legumes reduced the risk of colorectal adenomas by 17%.
Heart disease	Intake of 100 g of legumes four times per week reduced the risk of ischemic heart disease by 14%.
Hypercholesterolemia	Legumes decreased total cholesterol level by 11.8 mg/dL and LDL cholesterol level by 8.0 mg/dL in patients with hypercholesterolemia.
Obesity	Legumes reduced the body weight by 0.75 lb.
Prostate cancer	Legumes reduced the risk of prostate cancer by 15%.
	Daily intake of 20 g of legumes reduced the risk of prostate cancer by 3.5%.

• Recommendation

Prevention — For people at risk of chronic disease: men should consume ½ cup of cooked legumes, three times per week, and women should consume ½ cup of cooked legumes, three times per week.

Treatment — For chronic disease patients: men should consume ½ cup of cooked legumes, five times per week, and women should consume ½ cup of cooked legumes, four times per week.

Materials: Depending on the season, you may select legumes, such as black beans, green beans, lentils, kidney beans, chickpeas, lima beans, and the like. One half cup of cooked lentils is about 99 grams.

18

Low Salt

About 200,000 years ago, the human's salt intake was approximately 0.1–0.5 g per day, which was like the intake of the great apes. During the hunter-gatherer era, salt intake was still less than 1 g per day. In 6000 BCE, in the Shanxi region of China, people harvested salt deposits from the surface of dried lakes during hot summer months. In the following millennia, salt was used as a condiment, and to cure and preserve foods, and the human's salt intake increased to about 5 to 9 g per day. After WW II, refrigerators replaced salt as the primary way to preserve food. In theory, people's daily salt intake should have decreased, but the data shows otherwise. The main reason was the availability of processed foods and fast foods, most of which contain high salt. Starting from the 1950s, the daily lives and activities of Americans became busier, and people did not have time to prepare home meals, so they began relying on ready-to-eat meals, such as processed food and fast food. The high-salt content of processed foods and fast foods are at least partly responsible for the average daily intake of 12 g of salt per capita in the United States. The World Health Organization recommends that a person's daily salt intake should not exceed 6 g (or 2.3 g sodium).

Although salt *per se* has no antioxidant potential, high salt intake is known to suppress renal cortical expression of antioxidant enzymes, such as superoxide dismutase, and increase oxidative stress in the kidneys, vascular system, and other organs. Contrary to that, low salt intake facilitates expression of antioxidant enzymes and provides protection against free radical damage in the body.

What Types of Chronic Disease can be Prevented by Low Salt Intake?

• Meta-analysis

Hypertension — A daily intake of low salt (4.4 g) can significantly lower blood pressure in both child and adult hypertensive patients.

A meta-analysis of thirty-seven double-blind randomized clinical trials in adults and nine double-blind randomized clinical trials in children examined the association between salt intake and hypertension found that restriction of salt intake to 6 g per day decreased systolic pressure by 3.47 mmHg and diastolic pressure by 1.54 mmHg in adult hypertensive patients and decreased systolic pressure by 0.84 mmHg and diastolic pressure by 0.87 mmHg in child hypertensive patients. In addition, reduction in salt intake led to lower risks of stroke and fatal coronary heart disease in adult hypertensive patients. No adverse effect was observed on blood lipids, catecholamine levels, or renal function. Analysis confirms that restriction of salt intake to 6 g per day can noticeably lower blood pressure in hypertensive patients. Additional supporting evidence about the benefits of low salt is documented in a meta-analysis of 34 double-blind randomized clinical trials, which showed that daily intake of 4.4 g of salt for 4 weeks decreased systolic pressure by systolic pressure by 5.39 mmHg and diastolic pressure by 2.82 mmHg in hypertensive patients.

• Conclusion

Adult hypertensive patients who consumed 6 g of salt daily decreased systolic pressure by 3.5 mmHg and diastolic pressure by 1.5 mmHg, and child hypertensive patients who consumed 6 g of salt daily decreased systolic pressure by 0.8 mmHg and diastolic pressure by 0.9 mmHg (see Table 18.1). In addition, hypertensive patients who consumed 4.4 g of salt daily for 4 weeks decreased systolic pressure by 5.4 mmHg and diastolic pressure by 2.8 mmHg. The results support the prevailing view that daily intake of 4 to 6 g of salt can reduce blood pressure in patients with hypertension. Restricting daily salt intake to 6 g should be included in dietary recommendations for the prevention and management of hypertension.

Table 18.1.   Meta-analytical Confirmation of Low Salt Intake with Reduced Blood Pressure in Patients with Hypertension

Chronic Disease	Reduced Risk, Low Salt
Hypertension	Adult hypertensive patients who consumed 6 g of salt per day decreased systolic pressure by 3.5 mmHg and diastolic pressure by 1.5 mmHg.
	Child hypertensive patients who consumed 6 g of salt per day decreased systolic pressure by 0.8 mmHg and diastolic pressure by 0.9 mmHg.
	Hypertensive patients who consumed 4.4 g of salt per day for 4 weeks decreased systolic pressure by 5.4 mmHg and diastolic pressure by 2.8 mmHg.

• Recommendation

Prevention — For people at risk of hypertension: the recommended intake is 1 teaspoon of salt per day (or 6 g of salt per day).

Treatment — For hypertensive patients: the recommended intake is ½ teaspoon of salt per day (or 3–4 g of salt per day).

Material: Various salt products are available in the grocery stores in the United States. Select pure sea salt without additives. Read the food labels to determine your daily salt intake from the foods.

19

Milk

Not long ago, milk was an integral part of the traditional American breakfast. Most Americans enjoyed cereals with milk as part of their breakfast. Coming home from school, the first thing children did was to pull a glass of milk from the refrigerator. Now, the first thing children do after coming home from school is to grab a can of soda from the same refrigerator. According to the data from the USDA, the consumption of milk in the country reduced by 37% from 1970 to the present; milk has been replaced with increased consumption of coffee, fruit juices, and soda.

Human breast milk contains lactose. From birth until 5 years old, every infant and child on Earth can digest lactose in breast milk. After the age of 5, about 90% of all Eastern Asians, including Chinese, Japanese, Korean, Taiwanese, and South Eastern Asians lose their ability to digest lactose, which is called lactose intolerance. People who have lactose intolerance cannot digest lactose in foods such as milk. Incidental lactose intake can lead to flatulence, abdominal pain, and diarrhea. In contrast, about 90% of all Northern Europeans, including Germans, Russians, Finnish, Swedish, and Norwegians maintain their abilities to digest lactose into their adulthood, which is called lactose persistence. People who are lactose persistent can digest lactose containing foods, such as milk, without any discomfort. In the American grocery stores, there are many lactose-free products, including lactose-free milk, which would allow people with lactose intolerance to enjoy drinking milk without the fear of ill effects.

How do people acquire lactose intolerance or lactose persistence? In the Agriculture Era, humans domesticated fruits and vegetables as well as cows and sheep. Historical records documented that in 7000 BCE, milk and cheese were staple foods for humans living in Central Europe. At the time, children who inherited lactose persistence genes from parents could digest lactose in milk and cheese and grew properly. On the other hand, children who did not inherit lactose persistence genes from parents could not digest lactose in milk and cheese and grew poorly. Over thousand years of natural selection and evolution, most Europeans have become lactose persistent. However, humans living in Asia regions did not domesticate milk cows or sheep in the Agriculture Era and did not have to rely on dairy products as staple foods; therefore, lactose persistence genes were suppressed, which resulted in lactose intolerance in most Asian populations.

French scientist Louis Pasteur was rightfully credited for popularizing global milk consumption. In 1863, Pasteur invented a low-temperature sterilization technique, which later was named pasteurization in honor of him. Pasteur found that simply heating milk to 72°C for 15 seconds was enough to kill all bacterial spores in raw milk, which gave rise to pasteurized milk that is nutritious and free of germs. Various kinds of milk are available in the grocery stores in the United States. Milk is often categorized based on its fat contents: whole milk (3.5% fat), low-fat milk (1–2% fat) and skim milk (less than 0.5% fat).

What are the major nutrients in milk?

Milk contains high amounts of nutrients including milk proteins, calcium, potassium, Vitamin A, Vitamin B2, Vitamin B3, Vitamin B9, Vitamin B12, and Vitamin D (see Table 19.1), all of which are beneficial to human health, including strengthening bone density and protecting the heart and vascular system. Furthermore, milk contains both water-soluble and fat-soluble antioxidants, which work synergistically to enhance antioxidant defense system to protect against free radical damage throughout the body.

Table 19.1. The Major Nutrients in Whole Milk

Nutrients	Unit	Amount, per 100 g	Nutrients	Unit	Amount, per 100 g
Water	G	88.13	Vitamin B1	Mg	0.046
Energy	Calorie	61	Vitamin B2	Mg	0.169
Protein	G	3.15	Vitamin B3	Mg	0.089
Total fat	G	3.25	Vitamin B6	Mg	0.036
Saturated fat	G	1.865	Vitamin B9	mcg	5
Monounsaturated fat	G	1.981	Vitamin B12	mcg	0.45
Polyunsaturated fat	g	0.195	Vitamin A	IU	46
Cholesterol	mg	10	Vitamin A	mcg	162
Sugar	g	5.05	Vitamin E	Mg	0.07
Calcium	mg	113	Vitamin D	IU	51
Potassium	mg	132	Vitamin K	mcg	0.3

The data adapted from the 2016 USDA sources.

What Types of Chronic Disease can be Prevented by Consuming Milk?

• Meta-analysis

Breast cancer — Women who consume low-fat milk daily have lower risk of breast cancer.

A meta-analysis of twenty-seven research articles investigated the relationship between milk consumption and breast cancer in 1,500,312 participants showed that daily consumption of 500 g of milk reduced the risk of breast cancer by 10%, and daily consumption of 400–500 g of milk reduced the risk of breast cancer by 6%. Daily consumption of low-fat milk decreased the risk of breast cancer by 15%. Asian women who consumed milk reduced the risk of breast cancer by 24%.

Cardiovascular disease — People who consume milk regularly diminish the risk of cardiovascular disease.

Twenty-two prospective studies evaluated the association between milk consumption and cardiovascular disease in 127,160 people found that milk consumption reduced the risk of cardiovascular disease by 12%.

Cognitive impairment — Elderly people who consume milk regularly can lower the risk of cognitive impairment, particularly in elderly Asians.

A meta-analysis of seven prospective studies evaluated the association between milk consumption and cognitive impairment in 10,941 people revealed that milk consumption reduced the risk of cognitive impairment by 28%. The effect was especially noticeable in the Asian population.

Colorectal cancer — Daily consumption of milk can significantly lower the risk of colorectal cancer, particularly in men.

Sixty epidemiological studies investigated the relationship between milk consumption and colorectal cancer including 26,335 colorectal cancer cases found that milk consumption reduced the risk of colorectal cancer by 22%. In brief, people who consume milk can bring down the risk of colorectal cancer. Another meta-analysis of nineteen prospective studies examined the association between milk intake and colorectal cancer revealed that a daily intake of 200 g of milk reduced the risk of colorectal cancer by 9%, which demonstrated that a daily consumption of 200 ml of milk curtailed the incidence of colorectal cancer. Further supporting evidence about the benefits of milk is documented in a meta-analysis of fifteen prospective studies in 900,000 people including 5,200 colorectal cancer cases, which showed that a daily consumption of 525 g of milk reduced the risk of colorectal cancer by 26% in men.

Hypertension — People who consume low-fat milk daily have lower risk of hypertension.

A meta-analysis of nine prospective studies investigated the relationship between milk consumption and hypertension in 57,257 people including 15,367 hypertensive cases found that daily consumption of 200 ml of low-fat milk decreased the risk of the incidence of hypertension by 4% in normotensive individuals. Whole milk, yogurt, or cheese was found to be less effective when compared to low-fat milk.

Obesity — Dairy consumption daily reduces the risk of obesity in both children and adults.

A meta-analysis of 33 prospective studies explored the association between dairy consumption and the risk of obesity found that dairy consumption reduced the risk of obesity in children and adults by 46% and 25%, respectively. In addition, milk consumption was found to lower the risk of obesity in children and adults by 17% and 23%, respectively. The dose-response analysis showed that each additional intake of 200 ml of milk per day decreased the risk of obesity by 16%.

Stroke — Daily intake of milk greatly lowers the incident rates of stroke.

Fifteen research articles examined the association between milk intake and stroke in 764,635 people including 28,138 stroke cases found that daily milk intake of 100 ml, 200 ml and 300 ml reduced the risk of stroke by 12%, 18% and 17%, respectively. Furthermore, daily milk intake of 400 ml, 500 ml, 600 ml, and 700 ml reduced the risk of stroke by 15%, 14%, 9% and 6%, respectively. A daily intake of 200–300 ml of milk provides the best protection against the incidence of stroke.

Type 2 diabetes — Consumption of low-fat milk (200 ml daily) curtails the risk of type 2 diabetes.

A meta-analysis of 14 prospective studies examined the relationship between milk consumption and type 2 diabetes in 426,055 participants, of which 26,976 were type 2 diabetes cases. The results showed that daily consumption of 200 ml of whole milk reduced the risk of type 2 diabetes by 2%, and daily consumption of 200 ml of low-fat milk reduced the risk of type 2 diabetes by 9%.

• Conclusion

The meta-analyses showed that consumption of milk reduced the risk of hypertension, cardiovascular disease, type 2 diabetes, stroke, breast cancer, colorectal cancer, and cognitive impairment (see Table 19.2). Milk consumption decreased the risk of hypertension,

Table 19.2. **Meta-analytical Confirmation of Milk Consumption Associated with Lower Risks of Chronic Diseases**

Chronic Diseases	Reduced Risk, Milk Consumption
Breast cancer	Daily consumption of low-fat milk reduced the risk of breast cancer by 15%.
	Daily intake of 400–500 ml and more than 500 ml of milk reduced the risk of breast cancer by 6% and 10%, respectively.
	Asian women who consumed milk daily reduced the risk of breast cancer by 24%.
Cardiovascular disease	Milk reduced the risk of cardiovascular disease by 12%.
Cognitive impairment	Milk reduced the risk of cognitive impairment by 28% in elderly people.
Colorectal cancer	Daily consumption of 200 ml of milk reduced the risk of colorectal cancer by 9%.
	Daily consumption of 525 ml of milk reduced the risk of colorectal cancer by 26% in men.
Hypertension	Daily consumption of 200 ml of low-fat milk reduced the risk of hypertension by 4% in normotensive individuals.
Obesity	Dairy foods reduced the risk of obesity in children and adults by 46% and 25%, respectively.
	Milk consumption reduced the risk of obesity in children and adults by 17% and 23%, respectively.
	Each additional consumption of 200 ml of milk decreased the risk of obesity by 16%.
Stroke	Daily consumption of 100 ml, 200 ml, 300 ml, 400 ml, 500 ml, 600 ml, and 700 ml of milk reduced the risk of stroke by 12%, 18%, 17%, 15%, 14%, 9%, 6%, respectively.
Type 2 diabetes	Daily intake of 200 ml of whole milk and 200 ml of low-fat milk reduced the risk of type 2 diabetes by 2% and 9%, respectively.

cardiovascular disease, and type 2 diabetes by 4%, 12%, and 9%, respectively. In addition, milk consumption reduced the risk of breast cancer by 15% and the risk of colorectal cancer by 22%. Milk consumption also reduced the risk of cognitive impairment by 28% in elderly people. Moreover, milk consumption reduced the risk of stroke by 18%. The milk consumption of 200 to 300 ml per day produces the best protection against the incidence of stroke.

In short, milk consumption is associated with lower risks of hypertension, cardiovascular disease, stroke, type 2 diabetes, and cognitive impairment as well as cancers, such as breast cancer and colorectal cancer. Incorporating milk into a healthy diet may prevent chronic diseases and cognitive impairment.

• **Recommendation**

Prevention — For people at risk of chronic disease: men should consume 300 ml of organic low-fat milk daily, and women should consume 200 ml of organic low-fat milk daily.

Treatment — For chronic disease patients: men should consume 400 ml of organic low-fat milk daily and women should consume 300 ml of organic low-fat milk daily.

Material: When purchasing, select organic low-fat milk, containing 1–2% milk fats. Organic milk is produced from cows that are not treated with antibiotics and growth hormones, and not fed with feeds made from animal parts.

20

Nuts

What are Nuts?

From the botanical viewpoint, nuts are actually fruits with hard outer shells. Yet, from a nutritional viewpoint, nuts refer to tree nuts, which include almonds, Brazil nuts, cashews, hazelnuts, macadamia nuts, walnuts, pistachios, pecans, and the like.

Have you ever wondered where nuts originated? The history of nuts is closely associated with the livelihoods of pre-historic humans. Nuts were nutritious and dependable foods for humans in the hunter-gather era. Recently, archeologists excavated an ancient site in Israel that dates back 780,000 years; among other artifacts, the site contained cracked nutshells and some intact nuts, including wild almond, water chestnut, acorn, and pistachio. The discovery provided direct evidence that nuts were staple foods for early homo sapiens.

Here is the brief history of five different kinds of tree nuts.

Walnuts — The walnut tree is perhaps the oldest tree on Earth. A recent archeological site in Iraq produced the first evidence of human consumption of wild walnuts about 50,000 years ago. In 2000 BCE, Babylonians (in the present-day Iraq) domesticated Persian walnut trees. In enduring millennia, Persian walnuts were the favorite food of the people living in the Mediterranean region, including the Greek and the Romans, and were used as offerings to gods. The black walnut tree is native to eastern North America. Walnut trees are grown commercially for timber and nuts.

Pecans — An archeological relic in Texas showed that in 6000 BCE, pecans were staple foods for native Americans during the autumn season. In the early 18th century, the Spaniards brought walnut trees from Texas to California, and now the State of California is one of the major pecan producing regions in the United States.

Pistachios — The pistachio tree was a native plant of Brazil. Pistachio trees prefer warm climate and can grow up to 50 feet tall. In the late 16th century, the Spaniards brought pistachio trees from Brazil to the Philippines, and subsequently pistachios spread across Asia.

Almonds — Almonds originated perhaps in China and Central Asia. During the medieval times, explorers recorded eating almonds along the "silk road" from Asia to the Mediterranean region such as Spain and Italy. In the 17th century, the Spaniards brought almond trees from Spain to California (at that time, a Spanish-occupied land). Now, almonds are one of the major crops in the State of California.

Macadamia nuts — In Hawaii, macadamia nuts are one of the local delicacies. In fact, the macadamia nut tree is a native plant in the rain forests of Queensland, Australia.

Brazil nuts — The Brazil nut tree is indigenous to the Amazon rain forests in Brazil. The original Brazil nut tree had nut pods, and each weighed 4 to 6 pounds and contained 15 to 30 Brazil nuts. To harvest, the local people had to climb the trees, cut the nut pods loose with machetes, and let them fall to the ground. The falling heavy nut pods could accidentally kill people who were standing near the trees.

Peanuts — From a botanical viewpoint, peanut is not a tree nut; rather, it is a legume. In 2000 BCE, the people in South America domesticated peanut plants, and in the 16th century, the Spaniards and the Portuguese brought peanut plants from South America to Africa, Europe, and the United States, and the peanut plant subsequently spread to the rest of the world.

What are the major nutrients in nuts?

Nuts are rich in antioxidant vitamins and essential elements. Table 20.1 illustrates the major nutrients of some common tree nuts. Among all tree nuts, almond contains the highest amount of calcium. Almond intake may strengthen bone density and reduce the risk of osteoporosis, particularly for people who cannot drink milk. Brazil nuts contain the highest amounts of selenium. Selenium enhances antioxidant and immune defenses and accelerates wound healing. You can fulfill your daily recommended intake of selenium just by eating two to three Brazil nuts. Cashews are an excellent source of iron. Iron, which is a required trace essential element for making hemoglobin, can also enhance antioxidant capacity and immune defense. Consumption of cashews may mitigate the condition in patients with iron insufficiency. In addition, hazelnuts contain the highest amount of Vitamin B9. Vitamin B9 or folic acid can protect the heart as well as improve memory and cognition. Macadamia nuts are rich in oleic acid, as well as magnesium, calcium, and potassium. If a cooking recipe calls for oily nuts, macadamia nuts would be your best choice. Pecans are excellent sources of dietary fiber and oleic acid, both of which can protect the cardiovascular system and lower the risk of heart disease and stroke. Lutein and zeaxanthin are potent antioxidants that can particularly protect the eyes and improve vision. Among all tree nuts, pistachio nuts contain the highest amount of lutein and zeaxanthin. Moreover, walnuts are an excellent plant source for omega-3 fatty acids. Omega-3 fatty acids can reduce cholesterol, protect the heart, and improve memory and brain health.

In addition, almonds and hazelnuts contain high amounts of Vitamin E (see Table 20.1). Vitamin E is an essential vitamin present in vegetables and nuts. It has a multitude of beneficial effects to health. First and foremost, Vitamin E is a strong antioxidant residing in the cell membrane of each cell, and it acts like a guard to get rid of any harmful free radicals and protect cell membrane from oxidative damage. The integrity of the cell membrane is essential for allowing the cells to produce energy and fulfill its metabolic functions.

Table 20.1. The Major Nutrients in Common Tree Nuts

Amount (1 ounce)	Almond	Brazil Nut	Cashew	Hazel Nut	Australian Nut	Pecan	Pistachio	Walnut
Calorie	163	186	157	178	204	196	159	185
Protein, g	6.0	4.1	5.2	4.2	2.2	2.6	5.8	4.3
Fat, g	14.0	18.8	12.4	17.2	21.5	20.4	12.9	18.5
Saturated fat, g	1.1	4.3	2.2	1.3	3.4	1.8	1.6	1.7
Polyunsaturated fat, g	3.4	5.8	2.2	2.2	0.4	6.1	3.9	13.4
Mono-unsaturated fat, g	8.8	7.0	6.7	12.9	16.7	11.6	6.8	2.5
Carbohydrate, g	6.1	3.5	8.6	4.7	3.9	3.9	7.8	3.9
Dietary fiber, g	3.5	2.1	0.9	2.7	2.4	2.7	2.9	1.9
Potassium, mg	200	187	187	193	104	116	291	125
Magnesium, mg	76	107	83	46	37	34	34	45
Zinc, mg	0.9	1.2	1.6	0.7	0.4	1.3	0.6	0.9
Copper, mg	0.3	0.5	0.6	0.5	0.2	0.3	0.4	0.5
Calcium, mg	75	45	10	32	24	20	30	28
Iron, mg	1.1	0.7	1.9	1.3	1.1	0.7	1.1	0.8
Vitamin B1, mg	1.0	0.1	0.3	0.5	0.7	0.3	0.4	0.3
Vitamin B9, mcg	14	6	7	32	3	6	14	28
Vitamin E, mg	7.35	1.63	0.26	4.27	0.16	0.40	0.55	0.51

The data adapted from the 2010 USDA sources.

Nuts are a relatively high calorie food, so some people worry that nut consumption may cause weight gain. However, consuming nuts will not cause weight gain because nuts contain concentrated amounts of dietary fiber and vegetable proteins, both of which can improve insulin sensitivity and help regulate glucose metabolism, which reduce the risk of obesity.

What Types of Chronic Disease can be Prevented by Consuming Nuts?

• Meta-analysis

Colorectal cancer — Regular consumption of nuts reduces the risk of colorectal cancer.

A meta-analysis of thirty-six prospective studies investigated the relationship between nut consumption and colorectal cancer including 30,708 colorectal cancer cases found that nut consumption reduced the risk of colorectal cancer by 24%.

Endometrial cancer — Women who regularly consume nuts have markedly lower risk of endometrial cancer.

Thirty-six research papers examined the association between nut intake and endometrial cancer revealed that consuming tree nuts reduced the risk of endometrial cancer by 42%.

Heart disease — Nut consumption profoundly curtails the incident rates of coronary heart disease.

A meta-analysis of 23 research articles evaluated the relationship between nut consumption and heart disease in 501,791 participants, of which 11,869 were ischemic heart disease cases, which showed that consumption of 28.5 g of mixed nuts 4 times a week decreased the risk of ischemic heart disease by 22%. In short, people who consume one ounce of nuts 4 times per week are found with lower risk of heart disease. Another meta-analysis of 123 prospective studies investigated the association of nut consumption and heart disease showed that nut consumption reduced the risk of coronary heart disease by 33%.

Hypercholesterolemia — Frequent consumption of nuts brings down blood cholesterol levels and favorably improves blood lipid profiles in hypercholesterolemic patients.

Sixty-one double-blind randomized clinical trials examined the relationship between nut intake and hypercholesterolemia found that daily consumption of 60 g of mixed nuts decreased the total cholesterol level by 4.7 mg/dL, LDL cholesterol level by 4.8 mg/dL, and triglycerides by 2.2 mg/dL in hypercholesterolemic patients. Analysis confirms that consumption of two ounces of mixed nuts per day significantly lowered blood cholesterol levels in hypertensive patients. Another meta-analysis of three double-blind randomized clinical trials evaluated the association between nut consumption and hypercholesterolemia revealed that daily consumption of 29–69 g of hazel nuts for 28 to 84 days decreased the total cholesterol level by 2.3 mg/dL and LDL cholesterol level by 2.7 mg/dL in hypercholesterolemic patients. In brief, a daily consumption of one to two ounces of hazel nuts favorably influences lipid and lipoproteins in patient with hypercholesterolemia. Further supporting evidence about the benefits of nuts is reported in the meta-analysis of 18 double-blind randomized clinical trials, which found that consumption of 43 g of almonds five times per week decreased the total cholesterol level by 2.8 mg/dL, LDL cholesterol level by 2.2 mg/dL and triglycerides by 1.2 mg/dL in hypercholesterolemic patients.

Hypertension — Regular consumption of nuts effectively lowers blood pressure in both pre-hypertensive individuals and hypertensive patients.

Nine research papers investigated the association between nut consumption and hypertension found that consuming more than two servings of nuts per week reduced the risk of hypertension by 8% in pre-hypertensive individuals. Interestingly, nut consumption of one serving per week was not found to be effective. Two servings of mixed nuts per week were effective in lowering the risk of hypertension. Another meta-analysis of 21 double-blind randomized clinical trials showed that nut consumption decreased systolic pressure by 1.3 mmHg in hypertensive patients. Further analysis revealed that consuming pistachios decreased systolic pressure by 1.8 mmHg and diastolic pressure by 0.8 mmHg in pre-diabetic hypertensive patients.

Pancreatic cancer — Frequent consumption of mixed nuts greatly reduces the risk of pancreatic cancer.

A meta-analysis studied the association between nut consumption and pancreatic cancer revealed that nut consumption reduced the risk of pancreatic cancer by 32%.

Premature mortality — Regular consumption of tree nuts can prevent premature mortality, including all-cause, neurodegenerative disease, cardiovascular disease, cancer, and respiratory disease mortalities.

Fifteen research articles examined the relationship between nut consumption and premature mortality in 354,636 participants, of which 44,636 were mortality cases. The results showed that consumption of one serving of mixed nuts per week reduced the risk of all-cause mortality by 4% and the risk of cardiovascular disease mortality by 7%. In addition, daily consumption of one serving of mixed nuts reduced the risk of all-cause mortality by 27% and the risk of cardiovascular disease mortality by 39%. The results confirm that daily consumption of mixed nuts can reduce the risk of premature mortality. Another meta-analysis evaluated the relationship between nut consumption and premature mortality in 120,852 people including 8,823 mortality cases found that nut consumption in the amounts of 1–5 g, 5–10 g, and greater than 10 g per day reduced the risks of all-cause mortality by 12%, 26%, and 23%, respectively. The dose-response studies showed that a daily intake of 10 g of nuts reduced the risk of neurodegenerative disease mortality, cardiovascular disease mortality, cancer mortality, and respiratory disease mortality by 44%, 17%, 15%, and 29%, respectively. The analysis demonstrates that daily consumption of one-half ounce of mixed nuts can reduce the incidence of all-cause mortality as well as disease-specific mortalities, including mortalities from neurodegenerative disease, cardiovascular disease, cancer, and respiratory disease. Additional supporting evidence about the benefits of nuts, a meta-analysis of 28 research papers in 819,448 people revealed that a daily consumption of 28 g of nuts reduced the risk of all-cause mortality, respiratory disease mortality, type 2 diabetes mortality, neurodegenerative disease mortality, infectious disease mortality, and kidney disease mortality by 28%, 52%, 39%, 35%, 75%, and 73%, respectively. The studies claimed that insufficient consumption of tree nuts led to 4.4 million people died prematurely each year in the United States, Europe, Eastern Asia, and Western Pacific regions.

Stroke — Consumption of mixed nuts (one-half ounce daily) significantly lowers the risk of incident stroke.

A meta-analysis of 14 research papers evaluated the association between nut consumption and stroke found that nut consumption reduced the risk of stroke by 12% in men and the risk of stroke by 16% in women. In addition, a daily intake of 12 g of mixed nuts reduced the risk of stroke by 14%.

Type 2 diabetes — Consumption of mixed nuts (two ounces daily) decreases the fasting glucose level and ameliorates the condition of the disease in patients with type 2 diabetes.

Twelve double-blind randomized clinical trials investigated the relationship between nut consumption and type 2 diabetes showed that daily consumption of 56 g of mixed nuts decreased the fasting glucose level by 2.7 mg/dL in type 2 diabetic patients.

• Conclusion

The meta-analytical data in Table 20.2 illustrates that nut consumption reduced hypertension, hypercholesterolemia, type 2 diabetes, heart disease, stroke, endometrial cancer, pancreatic cancer, and colorectal cancer. People who regularly consumed nuts were found to lower the risk of hypertension by 8%. In addition, consumption of nuts reduced the total cholesterol level by 4.7 mg/dL, LDL cholesterol level by 4.8 mg/dL, and triglycerides by 2.2 mg/dL in hypercholesterolemic patients. For men, nut consumption decreased the risk of stroke by 12% and for women, nut consumption decreased the risk of stroke by 16% and the risk of endometrial cancer by 42%. Consumption of nuts is also shown to reduce the

Table 20.2.   Meta-analytical Confirmation of Nut Consumption Associated with Lower Risks of Chronic Diseases as well as Premature Mortality

Chronic Diseases	Reduced Risk, Nut Consumption
Colorectal cancer	Daily intake of nuts reduced the risk of colorectal cancer by 24%.
Endometrial cancer	Daily intake of nuts reduced the risk of endometrial cancer by 42%.
Heart disease	Intake of 28.5 g of nuts four times per week reduced the risk of ischemic heart disease by 22%.
Hypercholesterolemia	Daily consumption of 60 g of mixed nuts decreased total cholesterol level by 4.7 mg/dL, LDL cholesterol level by 4.8 mg/dL, and triglycerides by 2.2 mg/dL in hypercholesterolemic patients.
	Daily consumption of 29–69 g of hazel nuts for 28 to 84 days decreased total cholesterol level by 2.3 mg/dL and LDL cholesterol level by 2.7 mg/dL in hypercholesterolemic patients.
	Consumption of 43 g of almonds five times per week decreased total cholesterol level by 2.8 mg/dL, LDL cholesterol level by 2.2 mg/dL, and triglycerides by 1.2 mg/dL in hypercholesterolemic patients.
Hypertension	Nuts reduced the risk of hypertension by 8% in pre-hypertensive individuals.
	Nuts decreased systolic pressure by 1.3 mg/dL in hypertensive patients.
Pancreatic cancer	Nuts reduced the risk of pancreatic cancer by 32%.
Premature mortality	One serving of nuts per week reduced the risk of all-cause mortality and cardiovascular mortality by 4% and 7%, respectively.
	One serving of nuts per day reduced the risk of all-cause mortality, respiratory disease mortality, type 2 diabetes mortality, neurodegenerative disease mortality, infectious disease mortality, and kidney disease mortality by 28%, 52%, 39%, 35%, 75%, and 73%, respectively.
Stroke	Nuts reduced the risk of stroke in men and women by 12% and 16%, respectively.
Type 2 diabetes	Intake of 56 g of mixed nuts per day decreased fasting glucose level by 2.7 mg/dL in type 2 diabetic patients.

risk of pancreatic cancer by 32% and the risk of colorectal cancer by 24%. Moreover, the meta-analytical data showed that consumption of one serving of nuts per day lowered the risk of premature mortality, including the risk of all-cause mortality, cardiovascular mortality, and neurodegenerative disease mortality by 28%, 17%, and 35%, respectively. In addition, consumption of one serving of nuts per day also reduced the risk of respiratory disease mortality, infectious disease mortality, and kidney disease mortality by 52%, 75%, and 73%, respectively.

In conclusion, the meta-analytical results have demonstrated that nut consumption can improve blood lipid profiles in hypercholesterolemic patients, reduce blood pressure in hypertensive patients, and lower the fasting glucose levels in type 2 diabetic patients. Nut consumption is also associated with lower risks of type 2 diabetes, cardiovascular diseases, gastrointestinal cancers, and gynecological cancers as well as premature mortality. Incorporating nuts as a part of a healthy diet may prevent chronic diseases and help you live a longer life.

• **Recommendation**

Prevention — For people at risk of chronic diseases: men should consume one quarter cup of mixed nuts three times per week, and women should consume one quarter cup of mixed nuts two times per week.

Treatment — For chronic disease patients: men should consume one quarter cup of mixed nuts five times per week, and women should consume ¼ cup of mixed nuts three times per week.

Materials: Select mixed nuts contain at least almonds, walnuts, pistachios, cashews, and Brazil nuts. One-quarter cup of mixed nuts is about 31 g.

21

Olive Oil

In recent years, the American bookstore shelves display a dazzling array of diet related books. Among all diet books, the Mediterranean diet is still the most popular healthy diet. It mainly consists of vegetables, fruits, whole grains, legumes, olive oil, fish, and chicken. The average American consumes about one liter of olive oil per capita per year, while the average olive oil consumption of Greek, Italian, and Spaniard per capita per year is about 13 liters. There is a striking 13-fold difference between Americans and Europeans in annual olive oil consumption. Scientists speculate that such large difference in olive oil consumption might be a contributing factor for lower incident rates of heart diseases in Europeans compared to Americans.

Where did the olive tree come from?

The olive tree is a native plant of Asia Minor (now Turkey). About 6,000 years ago, olive tree cultivation spread from Asia Minor to Iraq, Syria, and Palestine and then to all Mediterranean regions. Olive oil is extracted from olives and has many beneficial uses. Olive oil can be used for cooking, in oil lamps at religious ceremonies, and even for skin care. In Roman times, people liked to moisturize their skin with olive oil after baths. For thousands of years, olive oil has been a quintessential ingredient of the Mediterranean diet. Most of the olive oil are triglycerides made of oleic acid and glycerol, although it may contain small amounts of free oleic acid, palmitic acid, and other fatty acids. Higher quality of olive oil generally has a lower content of free fatty acids. Virgin olive oil means olive oil that is produced by mechanically crushing olives and extracting the oil from the juice without subjecting it to any chemical treatment. However, over 50% of olive oil produced from the Mediterranean region is of poor quality and even not edible. The crude olive oil is treated via a chemical treatment process using charcoal and other chemicals to produce refined olive oil that is tasteless, odorless and colorless. To enhance its flavor, refined olive oil usually contains 10% to 15% of extra virgin olive oil. Extra virgin olive oil is the highest quality of olive oil with a least amount of free fatty acid and a pleasant flavor of fresh olives.

According to the 2010 USDA guidelines, olive oil can be categorized into at least four different grades.

- US Extra Virgin Olive Oil — The highest quality olive oil contains less than 0.8 g of free fatty acids per 100 g olive oil (0.8%).
- US Virgin Olive Oil — A good quality olive oil contains less than 2 g of free fatty acids per 100 g of olive oil (2%).
- US Olive Oil — A fair quality olive oil that contains a blend of 85% of refined olive oil and 15% of virgin olive oil.
- US Refined Olive Oil — Common olive oil produced by charcoal and other chemical filtration treatment.

Refined olive oil is suitable for baking or cooking purposes, while virgin olive oil and extra virgin olive oil can be used as a condiment such as salad dressing. Cooking at high temperature might destroy the flavor in olive oil. To maintain the flavor of olives, cooking temperature should not be higher than 216°C (or 421°F). Selecting the right extra virgin olive oil or virgin olive oil for your food is like selecting the right wine to match the food. By trial and error, you will eventually find your favorite olive oil and further enhance your salacious palate and dining experience.

Table 21.1.   The Major Nutrients in Virgin Olive Oil

Nutrients	Unit	14 g (or 1 teaspoon)	100 g
Energy	Calorie	130	929
Protein	g	0	0
Carbohydrate	g	0	0
Essential element Sodium	mg	0	0
Total fat	g	14	100
Saturated fat		2.001	14.290
Monounsaturated fat		10.00	71.430
Polyunsaturated fat		2.001	14.290
Trans fat		0	0
Cholesterol		0	0

The data adapted from the 2017 USDA sources.

What are the major nutrients in olive oil?

Understandably, people are generally afraid of too much oil or fat in their foods, particularly animal fats. Olive oil is nonetheless the healthiest dietary oil available in the world. Table 21.1 depicts the major nutrients in virgin olive oil, which has a high amount of monounsaturated fatty acids such as oleic acid and contains no cholesterol. 10 g of olive oil has 7.1 g of monounsaturated fatty acids, 1.4 g of polyunsaturated fatty acids, and 1.4 g of saturated fatty acids. To maintain good health, our bodies need monounsaturated fatty acids and polyunsaturated fatty acids, but they also require some saturated fatty acids. In addition to fatty acids, olive oil is an excellent food source of antioxidant Vitamin E and Vitamin K.

What are the benefits of consuming olive oil?

Olive oil contains high levels of polyphenols, of which 80% are oleuropein. The antioxidant oleuropein can neutralize free radicals, inhibit the oxidation of LDL cholesterol, decrease blood glucose level, prevent atherosclerosis, and reduce the risk of cardiovascular disease, stroke and type 2 diabetes. Among all vegetable oils, olive oil is the best oil available for the protection against the incidence of cardiovascular disease.

What Types of Chronic Disease can be Prevented by Consuming Olive Oil?

• Meta-analysis

Cardiovascular disease — People who regularly consume olive oil have a lower risk of cardiovascular disease.

Forty-two research papers investigated the relationship between olive oil intake and cardiovascular disease in 841,211 people found that olive oil intake reduced the risk of cardiovascular disease by 9%.

Stroke — Regular consumption of olive oil can noticeably lower the risk of stroke.

A meta-analysis of thirty-two prospective studies examined the association between olive oil consumption and stroke showed that consumption of olive oil reduced the risk of stroke by 17%.

Type 2 diabetes — Olive oil intake decreases the fasting glucose levels in both pre-diabetic individuals and type 2 diabetic patients, and mitigates the condition of the disease in patients with type 2 diabetes.

Twenty-nine double-blind randomized clinical trials evaluated the relationship between olive oil consumption and type 2 diabetes found that consumption of olive oil decreased the fasting glucose level by 8 mg/dL and HbA1c by 0.27% in type 2 diabetic patients. Consuming olive oil was also found to reduce the risk of type 2 diabetes by 16% in pre-diabetic individuals. In addition, daily consumption of 10 g of olive oil reduced the risk of type 2 diabetes by 9%.

• Conclusion

The meta-analytic data in Table 21.2 illustrates that regular olive oil consumption reduced the risk of cardiovascular disease, stroke, and type 2 diabetes. People who consumed olive oil reduced the risk of cardiovascular disease by 9%, the risk of type 2 diabetes by

Table 21.2. Meta-analytic Confirmation of Olive Oil Intake Associated with Lower Risks of Chronic Diseases

Chronic Diseases	Reduced Risk, Olive Oil
Cardiovascular disease	Olive oil reduced the risk of cardiovascular disease by 9%.
Stroke	Olive oil reduced the risk of stroke by 17%.
Type 2 diabetes	Olive oil reduced the risk of type 2 diabetes by 16% in pre-diabetic individuals. Daily intake of 10 g of olive oil reduced the risk of type 2 diabetes by 9%. Olive oil decreased fasting glucose level by 8 mg/dL and HbA1c by 0.27% in patients with type 2 diabetes.

16%, and the risk of stroke by 17%. Consumption of olive oil could also lower the fasting glucose level in patients with type 2 diabetes. In brief, consumption of olive oil may prevent cardiovascular disease and type 2 diabetes and may also mitigate the condition of the disease in patients with type 2 diabetes. It is recommended that olive oil should be included as part of a healthy diet to prevent and treat chronic diseases.

• Recommendation

Prevention — For people at risk of chronic diseases: men should consume one teaspoon of virgin olive oil three times per day, and women should consume one teaspoon of virgin olive oil twice per day.

Treatment — For chronic disease patients: men should consume 1½ teaspoon of virgin olive oil three times per day, and women should consume one teaspoon of virgin olive oil three times per day.

Material: Select either virgin olive oil or extra virgin olive oil. One teaspoon of virgin olive oil is about 14 g.

22

Pomegranate

The pomegranate tree is a native plant of Iran, Afghanistan and Pakistan, and it has been successfully cultivated throughout the Mediterranean region, Asia, Africa, and Europe, since the dawn of human civilization. For thousands of years, the tree bark, root, fruit, and peel of pomegranates have been used for medicinal applications. Pomegranates contain abundant amounts of antioxidant polyphenols, which can neutralize free radicals, mitigate free-radical induced damage, protect the cardiovascular system, and prevent atherosclerosis and hypertension. In addition, pomegranates are excellent food sources of Vitamin C, which can also protect the heart and vascular system while reducing the risk of hypertension.

What Types of Chronic Disease can be Prevented by Consuming Pomegranate Juice?

• Meta-analysis

Hypertension — Daily intake of pomegranate juice can significantly lower blood pressure in hypertensive patients.

Eight double-blind randomized clinical trials investigated the relationship between consumption of pomegranate juice and hypertension found that a daily intake of 240 ml pomegranate juice decreased systolic pressure by 5.0 mmHg and diastolic pressure by 2.0 mmHg in hypertensive patients. Interestingly, further studies revealed that a daily intake of less than 240 ml led to a more dramatic decrease in systolic pressure by 11.0 mmHg, while a daily intake of more than 240 ml only decreased systolic pressure by 3.6 mmHg. Daily intake of 100–200 ml of pomegranate juice was found to greatly improve blood pressure in hypertensive patients, and a daily intake of more than 240 ml was less effective.

• Conclusion

Pomegranate juice intake greatly decreased blood pressure in hypertensive patients as shown in Table 22.1. Interestingly, the degree to which blood pressure was reduced seemed relative to the amount of daily pomegranate consumption, but more consumption did not produce more dramatic decreases. A daily intake of 240 ml of pomegranate juice decreased systolic pressure by 5 mmHg and diastolic pressure by 2 mmHg. However, reducing the quantity of pomegranate juice consumed produced better results for reducing blood pressure. When the daily intake was reduced to between 100 to 200 ml of pomegranate juice, hypertensive patients experienced an 11 mmHg decrease in systolic pressure. Increasing the daily intake to more than 240 ml of pomegranate juice only decreased systolic pressure by 4 mmHg. In short, the optimal amount of pomegranate juice to produce the best result in controlling blood pressure of hypertensive patients appears to be between 100 to 200 ml per day. Pomegranate juice should be considered a safe and effective food remedy to prevent and treat hypertension.

Table 22.1. Meta-analytical Confirmation of Pomegranate Juice Intake Associated with a Lower Risk of Hypertension

Chronic Disease	Reduced Risk, Pomegranate Juice
Hypertension	Daily consumption of 240 ml of pomegranate juice decreased systolic pressure by 5.0 mmHg and diastolic pressure by 2.0 mmHg in hypertensive patients. Daily consumption of 100–200 ml of pomegranate juice decreased systolic pressure by 11.0 mmHg in hypertensive patients.

- ## Recommendation

Prevention — For people at risk of hypertension: men should drink 6 ounces of pure pomegranate juice each day, and women should drink 4 ounces of pure pomegranate juice each day.

Treatment — For hypertensive patients: men should drink 7 ounces of pure pomegranate juice each day, and women should drink 5 ounces of pure pomegranate juice a day.

Materials: When purchasing, select organic pomegranate juice with no added sugar. You can also buy whole pomegranates and prepare the juice at home using a fruit blender. Ripe pomegranates are in dark red color. A darker red pomegranate indicates that the fruit will be sweeter. Do not consume more than 10 ounces of pomegranate juice per day.

23

Probiotics

Probiotics are beneficial bacteria that are commonly added to food items, such as yogurt and other dairy foods, to improve the gut health. From head to toe, the human body hosts about 10 trillion of bacteria and contains only 1 trillion of cells. In other words, the number of bacteria living symbiotically with us are 10 times more than our own cells. Needless to say, bacteria are ubiquitous in our eyes, ears, mouth, armpits, skin, and the entire digestive tract. Bacteria are crucial for our gut health. In the digestive tract, beneficial bacteria include bifidobacteria and lactobacilli, and harmful bacteria include enterococci and *Escherichia coli*. In a healthy individual, the digestive tract is predominantly occupied by beneficial bacteria. However, in a type 2 diabetic patient, the digestive tract is dominated by harmful bacteria. Harmful bacteria can release lipopolysaccharides, antigens that can trigger inflammation, diminish insulin production in the pancreas, raise blood glucose level, and increase the risk of type 2 diabetes. In addition, antioxidant properties of probiotics, through probiotic bacteria, can boost antioxidant defense functions in the gut. Replenishing the digestive tract with beneficial bacteria in probiotics can decrease fasting glucose level, mitigate insulin resistance, and reduce the risk of type 2 diabetes.

What Types of Chronic Disease can be Prevented by Consuming Probiotics?

• Meta-analysis

Hypercholesterolemia — Regular intake of probiotics can favorably influence blood cholesterol levels in type 2 diabetic patients.

Twelve double-blind randomized clinical trials studied the relationship between probiotics and hypercholesterolemia found that probiotics consumption increased the HDL cholesterol level by 7.6 mg/dL, but had no discernible effect on the levels of LDL cholesterol, total cholesterol, or triglycerides in type 2 diabetic patients.

Type 2 diabetes — Regular consumption of probiotics can lower blood glucose levels in type 2 diabetic patients.

A meta-analysis of eleven double-blind randomized clinical trials evaluated the association between probiotics and type 2 diabetes showed that consumption of probiotics decreased the fasting glucose level by 9.5 mg/dL and HbA1c by 0.32% in type 2 diabetic patients.

• Conclusion

The meta-analytical results showed that consumption of probiotics decreased the fasting glucose level and hemoglobin A1c in patients with type 2 diabetes (see Table 23.1). Probiotics intake decreased fasting glucose level by 9.5 mg/dL and hemoglobin A1c by 0.32% as well as increased HDL cholesterol by 7.6 mg/dL in patients with type 2 diabetes. The results support the view that probiotics are effective in glycemic control of type 2 diabetes and should be implemented in dietary recommendations in the care and management of patients with type 2 diabetes.

Table 23.1. Meta-analytical Confirmation of Probiotics Associated with Reduced the Condition in Patients with Type 2 Diabetes

Chronic Diseases	Reduced Risk, Probiotics
Hypercholesterolemia	Probiotics increased HDL cholesterol level by 7.6 mg/dL in type 2 diabetic patients.
Type 2 diabetes	Probiotics decreased fasting glucose by 9.5 mg/dL and HbA1C by 0.32% in patients with type 2 diabetes.

• Recommendation

Prevention — For people at risk of type 2 diabetes: the recommended intake for men is 3 ounces of probiotics yogurt each day, and the recommended intake for women is 2 ounces of probiotics yogurt each day.

Treatment — For type 2 diabetic patients: the recommended intake for men is 2 ounces of probiotics yogurt twice each day, and the recommended intake for women is 3 ounces of probiotics yogurt each day.

Material: Select low sugar and unflavored probiotic yogurt. One cup of 8 ounces of probiotic yogurt typically contains about 10–15 g of lactose.

24

Resveratrol

Scientists in Japan first reported the isolation of resveratrol from the root of the *Veratrum album* in 1939. Resveratrol is also present in grapes, blueberries, and pomegranate. In grapes, resveratrol acts like a natural antibiotic and prevents the skin of grapes from bacterial and fungal infections during the ripening season. Resveratrol is a strong antioxidant that can quench free radicals and protect against oxidative damage to the vascular system, which may lead to hypertension.

What Types of Chronic Disease can be Prevented by Consuming Resveratrol?

- ## Meta-analysis

  Hypertension — Resveratrol supplement intake effectively reduces blood pressure in hypertensive patients.

  Six double-blind randomized clinical trials investigated the relationship between resveratrol and hypertension found that resveratrol at a dose of 150 mg per day reduced systolic blood pressure by 11.9 mmHg in hypertensive patients.

- ## Conclusion

  Resveratrol intake significantly reduced systolic blood pressure in hypertensive patients (see Table 24.1). The result supports the view that resveratrol should be included in dietary recommendations for the prevention and management of the incidence of hypertension.

Table 24.1. **Meta-analytical Confirmation of Resveratrol Associated with Reduced Blood Pressure in Patients with Hypertension**

Chronic Disease	Reduced Risk, Resveratrol
Hypertension	Daily intake of 150 mg of resveratrol decreased systolic pressure by 11.9 mmHg in hypertensive patients.

• Recommendation

Prevention — For people at risk of hypertension: the recommended dose for men is 500 mg of resveratrol supplement per day, and the recommended dose for women is 250 mg of resveratrol per day.

Treatment — For hypertensive patients: the recommended dose for men is 750 mg of resveratrol supplement per day, and the recommended dose for women is 500 mg of resveratrol supplement per day.

Material: Various resveratrol supplements are available in the marketplace. Select organic resveratrol supplement and take it with water before the bedtime. Avoid taking more than 2 g of resveratrol per day.

25

Rice Bran Oil

Rice originated in India. About 10,000 years ago, the Indians were among the first to cultivate rice, which then spread to China, Korea, Japan, Philippines, and Indonesia. In 327 BCE, Alexandra the Great and his armies invaded India and brought rice seeds back to the Mediterranean region, where the cultivation of rice quickly spread to Egypt, Spain, and Western Europe. In the mid-17th century, the Portuguese and the Dutch people managed large rice field plantations in West Africa and shipped harvested rice to North America via slave-trade voyages. The cultivation of rice in the United States therefore dates back to 400 years ago.

Rice bran oil is derived from the bran layer of a grain of rice, which has a concentrated content of linoleic acid. It is a widely used vegetable oil in Asian countries, such as Japan, China, and India. Since ancient times, rice bran oil has been used in brightening the complexion of the skin, accelerating wound healing, and repairing damaged hair. Linoleic acid can lower blood LDL cholesterol levels. In addition, unsaponifiable material (mostly lipids of natural origin) in rice bran oil has high antioxidant potential, which can hinder oxidative stress in the body, regulate the synthesis of cholesterol in the liver, and reduce blood cholesterol levels.

What Types of Chronic Disease can be Prevented by Consuming Rice Bran Oil?

• Meta-analysis

Hypercholesterolemia — Regular consumption of rice bran oil lowers blood cholesterol levels and favorably influences blood lipid and lipoproteins in patients with hypercholesterolemia.

A meta-analysis of eleven double-blind randomized clinical trials found that consumption of rice bran oil decreased the total cholesterol level by 12.7 mg/dL and the LDL cholesterol level by 6.9 mg/dL, and increased the HDL cholesterol level by 6.7 mg/dL in hypercholesterolemic patients.

• Conclusion

Consumption of rice bran oil decreased total cholesterol by 13 mg/dL and LDL cholesterol by 7 mg/dL and increased HDL cholesterol by 7 mg/dL in patients with hypercholesterolemia as shown in Table 25.1. The results provide compelling evidence that rice bran oil is effective in improving blood lipids and lipoproteins in patients with cholesterolemia. It is recommended that rice bran oil should be considered a safe and effective food remedy to prevent and treat patients with hypercholesterolemia.

Table 25.1. Meta-analytical Confirmation of Rice Bran Oil Associated with Favorably Improved Blood Lipid Profiles in Patients with Hypercholesterolemia

Chronic Disease	Reduced Risk, Rice Bran Oil
Hypercholesterolemia	Rice bran oil decreased total cholesterol level by 13 mg/dL and LDL cholesterol level by 7 mg/dL, and increased HDL cholesterol level by 7 mg/dL in patients with hypercholesterolemia.

• Recommendation

Prevention — For people at risk of hypercholesterolemia: men should consume one tablespoon of rice bran oil per day, and women should consume ½ tablespoon of rice bran oil per day.

Treatment — For hypercholesterolemic patients: men should consume two tablespoons of rice bran oil per day, and women should consume one tablespoon of rice bran oil per day.

Material: Select organic rice bran oil and mix it with cooked meals. One tablespoon of rice bran oil is about 13.6 g.

26

Soy Foods

Soybean originated in Southeast Asia regions. In 11,000 BCE, farmers in China domesticated soybeans. In subsequent millennia, China became the largest soybean producing country in the world. Soybean cultivation spread from China to Japan, Indonesia, Thailand, Malaysia, Vietnam, India, and Nepal between the 1st to 16th centuries. By 1910, China produced 87% of all soybeans in the world. American farmers began large-scale soybean production in the late 19th century and by 2000, farmers in the United States produced 55% of all soybeans in the world. Other major soybean producing countries include Brazil, China, India, and Argentina. However, soybeans produced in the United States are mainly used for agriculture animal feeds. Soy foods have been popular in Asia for centuries. Now, health conscious Americans and Europeans are embracing soy foods in their daily diets with foods, such as tofu and soy milk.

Dietary habits are known to influence incident rates of breast cancer and prostate cancer, and incident rates of these cancers vary among people who live in different countries. For instance, the incident rates of breast cancer and prostate cancer are lower in Japanese and Chinese populations compared to American and European populations. One major dietary difference between Asian countries and Western countries is the consumption of soy foods.

Soy foods contain isoflavones, such as genistein, daidzein, and equol. In the digestive tract, daidzein can be converted to equol, which has strong anti-cancer properties. However, owing to gene polymorphism, only 35% of people in the world can convert daidzein to equol in the digestive tract, and the conversion rate appears to be higher in Asians compared to Europeans. This disparity perhaps could explain why soy foods exhibit more anti-cancer activities in Asians, compared to Europeans. Genistein and daidzein, on the other hand, can inhibit the growth and proliferation of Helicobacter pylori bacteria residing in the stomach. The infestation and overgrowth of Helicobacter pylori bacteria is the known causative factor for the incidence of stomach cancer.

In addition, soy isoflavones and soy proteins, both of which can lower blood pressure in hypertensive patients. Blood flows through blood vessels transporting nutrients, oxygen, and water to cells everywhere in our bodies. The circulation system consists of arteries, veins, and capillaries. If all the blood vessels in the human body were linked together from end to end, they would stretch for about 60,000 miles! Proper elasticity and expandability of blood vessels is required to allow the blood to flow smoothly and continuously throughout the vast network of the circulatory system. To achieve that, the blood vessel constantly releases nitric oxide, a gaseous molecule and a potent vasodilator that supports and maintains the elasticity and expandability of the blood vessels. Insufficient nitric oxide levels in the bloodstream can lead to hypertension. Soy isoflavones support the synthesis of nitric oxide synthase enzyme in the blood vessels. Soy proteins contain a high amount of arginine, which is a substrate for nitric oxide synthase enzyme. Thus, soy foods can facilitate the release of nitric oxide from the blood vessels and prevent the incidence of hypertension.

Furthermore, soy isoflavones can inhibit the synthesis of cholesterol in the liver, and lower blood cholesterol level, and soy proteins decrease blood cholesterol level by stimulating the gallbladder to secrete cholesterol and bile juice. Soy proteins can also reduce hyperfiltration rates in diabetic patients with chronic kidney disease and assuage the progression and deterioration of renal functions in pre-dialysis chronic kidney disease patients.

Tofu is produced from soybean curd, like how cheese is produced from curds of milk proteins. Tofu contains an abundant number of nutrients, such as soy proteins, carbohydrates, lipids, isoflavones, and essential elements, such as calcium, magnesium, phosphorous, iron, manganese, and selenium. Tofu is an excellent protein source for vegetarians, particularly for those who prefer gluten-free foods.

What Types of Chronic Disease can be Prevented by Consuming Soy Foods?

• Meta-analysis

Breast cancer — Soy consumption lowers the risk of breast cancer in both pre- and postmenopausal women, and the risk of the recurrence of breast cancer in estrogen-positive breast cancer patients.

A meta-analysis of 15 research articles studied the relationship between soy consumption and breast cancer in 11,283 women found that the consumption of soy foods reduced the risk of breast cancer by 32%. Another meta-analysis of 61 prospective studies investigated the association between soy isoflavone intake and breast cancer showed that intake of soy isoflavone supplements reduced the risk of breast cancer in Asian women and Western women by 41% and 8%, respectively. The results confirm that soy isoflavone intake is effective in lowering the risk of breast cancer, particularly in Asian women. Further supporting evidence about the benefits of soy foods, a meta-analysis of five research papers evaluated soy consumption and breast cancer revealed that consumption of soy foods reduced the risk for the recurrence of breast cancer by 21%. In addition, consumption of soy foods reduced the risk of the recurrence of breast cancer by 28% in ER (estrogen receptor)-positive breast cancer patients. Moreover, consumption of soy foods reduced the risk of breast cancer in premenopausal and postmenopausal women by 22% and 19%, respectively.

Cardiovascular disease — Regular consumption of soy foods and/ or tofu brings down the risk of cardiovascular disease.

A meta-analysis of seventeen research papers examined the association between soy consumption and cardiovascular disease in 17,269 people found that consuming tofu reduced the risk of cardiovascular disease by 20%, and consuming soy foods reduced the risk of coronary heart disease by 17%.

Chronic kidney disease — Soy consumption decreases serum inflammatory markers and modestly improves the condition of the disease in patients with chronic kidney disease.

Nine double-blind randomized clinical trials investigated the relationship between soy protein intake and chronic kidney disease revealed that intake of soy proteins decreased serum creatinine level by 0.11 mg/dL and serum triglycerides by 4.1 mg/dL in pre-dialysis chronic kidney disease patients. In brief, soy consumption can ameliorate the condition of the disease in patients with chronic kidney disease. Another meta-analysis of twelve double-blind randomized clinical trials reported that intake of soy proteins decreased serum creatinine level by 0.05 mg/dL, serum phosphate level by 0.13 mg/dL, C-reactive protein by 0.98 mg/dL, and urine protein by 0.13 mg/day. The results further ascertain that soy protein intake can reduce serum creatinine, serum phosphate, and urine protein, and inflammatory mediators, such as C-reactive protein in chronic kidney disease patients. However, no significant change was found in creatinine clearance and glomerular filtration rate.

Colorectal cancer — Daily intake of soy foods and/or soy isoflavones can lower the risk of colorectal cancer.

A meta-analysis conducted by the United States Department of Agriculture found that women who habitually consumed soy foods reduced the risk of colorectal cancer by 21%. Analysis confirms that soy consumption can significantly lower the incidence of colorectal cancer. Another meta-analysis of forty research articles investigated the relationship between soy isoflavone intake and colorectal cancer in 633,476 people including 13,639 colorectal cancer cases showed that intake of soy isoflavones reduced the risk of colorectal cancer by 24%. In short, soy isoflavone intake is effective in reducing the risk of colorectal cancer. Additional supporting evidence about the benefits of soy isoflavones is documented in a meta-analysis of sixteen prospective studies, which showed that intake of soy isoflavone reduced the risk of colorectal cancer by 30%. The dose-response data revealed that each additional intake of 20 mg of soy isoflavones per day reduced the risk of colorectal cancer by 8%.

Endometrial cancer — Women who regularly consume soy foods have lower risks of endometrial cancers.

A meta-analysis of ten research articles examined the association between soy consumption and endometrial cancer found that soy consumption reduced the risk of endometrial cancer by 19%. In addition, soy consumption reduced the risk of endometrial cancer in Asian women and Western women by 21% and 17%, respectively. Moreover, soy consumption reduced the risk of endometrial cancer by 24% in postmenopausal women.

Heart disease — People who regularly consume soy foods have lower risks of coronary heart disease.

A meta-analysis of eleven research papers studied the relationship between soy consumption and heart disease including 7,616 coronary heart disease cases revealed that consuming soy foods reduced the risk of coronary heart disease by 34%.

Hypercholesterolemia — Daily intake of soy foods and/or soy proteins markedly lowers blood cholesterol levels and improves blood lipid profiles in patients with hypercholesterolemia.

Forty-three double-blind randomized clinical trials investigated the relationship between soy consumption and hypercholesterolemia revealed that daily intake of 15–30 g of soy foods decreased triglycerides by 10.7% and LDL cholesterol by 5.5%, and increased HDL cholesterol by 3.2%. Analysis demonstrates that daily consumption of one-half to one ounce of soy foods can significantly lower blood cholesterol levels in patients with hypercholesterolemia. Another meta-analysis of 35 double-blind randomized clinical trials investigated the relationship between soy consumption and hypercholesterolemia revealed that soy consumption decreased the total cholesterol level by 5.3 mg/dL, LDL cholesterol level by 4.8 mg/dL, and triglycerides by 4.9 mg/dL and increased the HDL cholesterol level by 1.4 mg/dL in patients with hypercholesterolemia. In other words, patients with hypercholesterolemia who regularly consume soy foods are found to favorably influence blood lipids and lipoproteins and assuaged the condition of the disease. Further supporting evidence about the benefits of soy foods, a meta-analysis of forty-two double-blind randomized clinical trials found that a daily consumption of 25 g of soy proteins decreased the total cholesterol level by 4.0 mg/dL, LDL cholesterol level by 4.2 mg/dL and triglycerides by 1.5 mg/dL in patients with hypercholesterolemia.

Hypertension — Daily intake of soy foods and/or soy isoflavones can lower blood pressure in both pre-hypertensive individuals and hypertensive patients.

Eleven double-blind randomized clinical trials investigated the relationship between soy consumption and hypertension reported that in pre-hypertensive individuals, soy consumption decreased systolic pressure by 2.5 mmHg and diastolic pressure by 1.5 mmHg. In hypertensive patients, soy consumption decreased systolic pressure by 5.9 mmHg and diastolic pressure by 3.4 mmHg. The results illustrate that soy consumption can lower blood pressure in hypertensive patients and pre-hypertensive individuals. Another meta-analysis of 14 double-blind randomized clinical trials evaluated the association between soy isoflavone intake and hypertension showed that a daily consumption of between 25 to 375 mg of soy isoflavones for 2 to 24 weeks decreased systolic pressure by 1.9 mmHg in hypertensive patients.

Lung cancer — Women who regularly consume soy foods have lower risk of lung cancer, particularly in non-smoking women.

Seven research articles examined the association between soy consumption and lung cancer in 71,550 women found that women who habitually consumed soy foods reduced the risk of lung cancer by 37%. The effect was especially noticeable in postmenopausal women. In addition, soy consumption reduced the risk of lung cancer in non-smoking women by 41%.

Obesity — Soy consumption daily leads to weight loss and lowers the risk of obesity.

A meta-analysis of three prospective studies evaluated the relationship between soy consumption and obesity in 133,468 people reported that each additional serving of soy foods daily reduced body weight by 2.47 lb.

Ovarian cancer — Women who regularly consume soy foods and/or soy isoflavones have lower risks of ovarian cancer.

A meta-analysis of seven research papers investigated the association between soy consumption and ovarian cancer showed that women who habitually consumed soy foods reduced the risk of ovarian cancer by 48% in pre- and postmenopausal women. Another meta-analysis of ten prospective studies examined the relationship between soy isoflavone intake and ovarian cancer revealed that intake of soy isoflavones reduced the risk of ovarian cancer by 30% in both pre-and postmenopausal women.

Prostate cancer — Soy consumption greatly curtails the risk of prostate cancer, particularly in Asian men.

Fifteen epidemiological studies investigated the relationship between soy foods and prostate cancer found that consumption of unfermented soy foods, such as tofu, reduced the risk of prostate cancer by 30% and consumption of fermented soy foods, such as natto, seemed to have no discernible effect. The results indicate that unfermented soy foods, such as tofu, can lower the risk of prostate cancer, and fermented soy foods, such as natto, are not effective. In addition, consumption of soy foods reduced the risk of prostate cancer by 48% in Asian men, but its effect was less obvious in Western men.

Stomach cancer — Consumption of unfermented soy foods, such as tofu and soy milk, decreases the risk of stomach cancer, while consumption of fermented soy foods, such as natto and miso, increases the risk of stomach cancer.

Twenty-two research articles examined the association between soy consumption and stomach cancer in 965,466 people including 12,901 stomach cancer cases found that soy consumption reduced the risk of stomach cancer by 15%, and for women, soy consumption reduced the risk of stomach cancer by 29%. Analysis demonstrates that regular consumption of soy foods can lower the risk of stomach cancer, particularly in women. Another meta-analysis of 38 research papers studied the relationship between soy foods and stomach cancer showed that soy consumption reduced the risk of stomach cancer by 36%. Contrary to that, consumption of fermented soy foods, such as natto and miso, was found to increase the risk of stomach cancer by 22%.

Stroke — People who frequently consume soy foods have lower risk of stroke.

A meta-analysis of five research articles investigated the association between soy consumption and stroke including 4,954 stroke cases revealed that soy consumption reduced the risk of stroke by 46%.

• Conclusion

As confirmed by the meta-analytical data, soy food consumption reduced the risk of hypertension, coronary heart disease, hypercholesterolemia, stroke, stomach cancer, lung cancer, breast cancer, endometrial cancer, ovarian cancer, prostate cancer, and colorectal cancer (see Table 26.1). Overweight or obese people who consumed soy foods lost an average of 2.47 lb, which suggests that consuming soy foods can promote weight loss in overweight and obese individuals. Consuming soy foods also reduced systolic pressure by 5.9 mmHg and diastolic pressure by 3.4 mmHg in hypertensive patients, which confirms that soy foods can help reduce blood pressure. In addition, soy consumption reduced triglycerides by 10.7% and LDL cholesterol level by 5.5%, and increased HDL cholesterol level by 3.2% in hypercholesterolemic patients. In short, consuming soy foods can promote weight loss in overweight

Table 26.1. Meta-analytical Confirmation of Soy Food Intake Associated with Lower Risks of Chronic Diseases

Chronic Diseases	Reduced Risk, Soy Foods
Breast cancer	Soy foods reduced the risk of breast cancer by 32%. Intake of soy isoflavones reduced the risk of breast cancer in Asian women and Western women by 41% and 8%, respectively. Soy foods reduced the risk of breast cancer recurrence by 21%.
Cardiovascular disease	Tofu reduced the risk of cardiovascular disease by 20%.
Chronic kidney disease	Soy proteins decreased serum creatinine, serum phosphate, serum triglycerides, urine protein, and C-reactive protein by 0.05–0.11 mg/dL, 0.13 mg/dL, 0.13 mg/day, 4.1 mg/dL, and 0.98 mg/dL, respectively.
Colorectal cancer	Soy consumption reduced the risk of colorectal cancer by 21%. Soy isoflavone supplement reduced the risk of colorectal cancer by 24–30%. Daily intake of 20 mg of soy isoflavones reduced the risk of colorectal cancer by 8%.
Endometrial cancer	Soy foods reduced the risk of endometrial cancer by 19%. Soy consumption reduced the risk of endometrial cancer in Asian women and Western women by 21% and 17%, respectively.
Heart disease	Soy foods reduced the risk of coronary heart disease by 34%.
Hypertension	Pre-hypertensive individuals who regularly consumed soy foods decreased systolic pressure by 2.5 mmHg and diastolic pressure by 1.5 mmHg. Hypertensive patients who regularly consumed soy foods decreased systolic pressure by 5.9 mmHg and diastolic pressure by 3.4 mmHg. Daily intake of 25–375 mg of soy isoflavones for 2 to 24 weeks decreased systolic pressure by 1.9 mmHg.
Hypercholesterolemia	Soy consumption decreased total cholesterol level by 5.3 mg/dL, LDL cholesterol level by 4.8 mg/dL, and triglycerides by 4.9 mg/dL, while it increased HDL cholesterol level by 1.4 mg/dL in patients with hypercholesterolemia.

Table 26.1. (*Continued*)

Chronic Diseases	Reduced Risk, Soy Foods
	Daily intake of 15–30 g of soy foods reduced LDL cholesterol level by 5.5% and triglycerides by 10.7%, and increased HDL cholesterol level by 3.2% in patients with hypercholesterolemia.
	Daily intake of 25 g of soy proteins decreased total cholesterol level by 4.0 mg/dL, LDL cholesterol level by 4.2 mg/dL, and triglycerides by 1.5 mg/dL in hypercholesterolemic patients.
Lung cancer	Women who regularly consumed soy foods reduced the risk of lung cancer by 37%.
	Non-smoking women who regularly consumed soy foods reduced the risk of lung cancer by 41%.
Obesity	Soy consumption reduced 2.47 lbs in weight.
Ovarian cancer	Women who regularly consumed soy foods reduced the risk of ovarian cancer by 48%.
Prostate cancer	Men who regularly consumed unfermented soy foods, such as tofu, reduced the risk of prostate cancer by 30%.
Stomach cancer	Soy consumption reduced the risk of stomach cancer by 15–36%.
Stroke	Soy consumption reduced the risk of stroke by 46%.

and obese individuals, reduce blood pressure in hypertensive patients, and improve blood cholesterol levels in patients with high blood cholesterol.

Moreover, the meta-analytical data revealed that consumption of soy foods reduced the risk of stroke by 46% and the risk of cardiovascular disease by 20%. The results demonstrate that consuming soy foods can protect the heart and vascular system and lower the risk of cardiovascular disease. Furthermore, soy foods reduced the risk of stomach cancer, lung cancer, and colorectal cancer by 15–36%, 37%, and 21%, respectively, which confirms the anti-cancer properties of soy foods. Soy isoflavones reduced the risk of breast cancer in Asian women and European women by 41% and 8%, respectively. Additionally, soy foods reduced the risk of endometrial cancer in Asian women and Western women by 21% and 17%, respectively. Postmenopausal women who consumed soy foods reduced the risk of endometrial cancer by 24% and the risk of ovarian cancer by 48%. Also, men who consumed soy foods reduced the risk of prostate cancer by 30%. Finally, consumption of soy foods has been found to improve the condition of patients with chronic kidney disease. Pre-dialysis chronic kidney disease patients and end-stage chronic kidney disease patients who consumed soy foods reduced serum creatinine, triglyceride levels, and phosphate levels, and decreased C-reactive protein and proteinuria.

The meta-analytic results provide convincing evidence that intake of soy foods is associated with lower risks of cardiovascular disease, chronic kidney disease, and many cancers. In brief, consuming soy foods promotes weight loss in overweight and obese individuals, lowers blood pressure in hypertensive patients, decreases blood cholesterol levels in hypercholesterolemic patients, reduces the risk of cardiovascular disease including coronary heart disease and stroke, and the risk of many cancers including breast cancer, endometrial cancer, ovarian cancer, and prostate cancer. Furthermore, soy food intake improves and maintains the remaining kidney functions in patients with chronic kidney disease. Instead of consuming animal proteins which can lead to proteinuria, patients with chronic kidney disease should consume soy foods to mitigate the problem with proteinuria as well as to improve the condition of the disease. People at risk of chronic diseases and chronic disease patients may want to consider including soy foods, such as soy milk and tofu, in a healthy nutrient-balanced diet.

• Recommendation for Soy Foods

Prevention — For people at risk of chronic diseases: men should consume ½ cup of cooked soy foods three times per week or drink 8 ounces of organic soy milk daily (no sugar added), and women should consume ½ cup of cooked soy foods, three times per week or drink 6 ounces of organic soy milk daily (no sugar added).

Treatment — For chronic disease patients: men should consume ½ cup of cooked soy foods five times per week or drink 10 ounces of organic soy milk daily (no sugar added), and women should consume ½ cup of cooked soy foods four times per week or drink 8 ounces of organic soy milk (no sugar added).

Material: Cooked soybeans are easy to prepare: add water to dry soybeans, heat it until boiling and simmer for 2 minutes. Select no sugar added organic soy milk. One-half cup of cooked soybeans is about 86 grams.

• Recommendation for Tofu

Prevention — For people at risk of cardiovascular disease: men should consume one-half cup of tofu three times per week, and women should consume one-half cup of tofu twice per week.

Treatment — For cardiovascular disease patients: men should consume one half cup of tofu five times per week, and women should consume one-half cup of tofu three times per week.

Materials: Two major kinds of tofu are soft tofu and firm tofu in the American grocery stores. Soft tofu is suitable for desserts and firm tofu is used mostly for cooking with other vegetables. One-half cup of tofu is about 4 ounces, which contains about 10 g of soy proteins.

27

Tomato

Around 700 CE, the Aztec people domesticated tomatoes in Central Mexico. In the mid-16th century, the Spaniards invaded Mexico and brought tomatoes back to Spain. Tomato cultivation soon became widespread in the Southern European countries. During the following century, many people in Europe died from eating tomatoes, and fear about tomato poisoning was rampant all over the Europe. The Europeans eschewed tomatoes because they believed tomatoes were poisonous. It was later discovered that tomato poisoning was due to the type of utensils that wealthy and royal families in Europe used, which were made from tin soldered with lead. The acids in tomato juice caused the lead to leach from the utensils into the cooked food. Tomato poisoning was in fact lead poisoning. Eating utensils in poor families were generally made from wood, which contained no lead, thus poor families incurred no incidences of tomato poisoning. Tomato then was a staple food only for poor families in Europe. In the 19th century, Italian immigrants brought pizzas to their newly adopted country. Americans began eating more tomatoes because of their love of pizza. Interestingly, tomato cultivation was not introduced to the United States from Mexico, the country where tomatoes originated; instead tomatoes detoured through Europe before arriving in the United States.

Tomatoes are an excellent food source of Vitamin C, Vitamin B6, Vitamin B9, and lycopene. Tomatoes also contain essential elements such as potassium, sodium, magnesium, and phosphate and essential trace elements such as iron, zinc, copper, and manganese.

The tomato's ability to prevent chronic diseases may be attributable to lycopene. Antioxidant lycopene can lower blood pressure, reduce blood levels of homocysteine, attenuate LDL cholesterol oxidation, and prevent platelet coagulation. Consumption of tomatoes helps maintain a healthy cardiovascular system and prevents cardiovascular disease. Lycopene can also interfere with growth factor receptor signaling and cell cycle progression in prostate cancer cells and reduce the risk of prostate cancer. Other possible anti-cancer mechanisms of lycopene include inhibition of inflammation, stimulation of xenobiotic metabolism in the liver, and reduce the risk of mutagenesis.

What Types of Chronic Disease can be Prevented by Consuming Tomatoes?

• Meta-analysis

Cardiovascular disease — Regular intake of lycopene supplement can lower the risk of cardiovascular disease.

Twenty-one clinical reports studied the relationship between lycopene consumption and hypertension found that lycopene supplement decreased systolic pressure by 5.7 mmHg in patients with cardiovascular disease.

Prostate cancer — Men who regularly consume tomatoes and/or take lycopene supplement have lower risk of prostate cancer.

Twenty-one research articles investigated the association between tomato consumption and prostate cancer found that consumption of raw tomato reduced the risk of prostate cancer by 11%, while consumption of cooked tomato reduced the risk of prostate cancer by 19%. The results confirm that elderly men who regularly consumed tomatoes can lower the risk of prostate cancer. Another meta-analysis of twenty-six research papers examined the relationship between lycopene intake and prostate cancer in 563,299 men including 17,517 prostate cancer cases showed that daily intake of 9–21 mg of lycopene supplement reduced the risk of prostate cancer by 21%.

• Conclusion

Table 27.1 illustrates that tomato consumption reduced systolic blood pressure by 5.7 mmHg in cardiovascular disease patients. In addition, men who regularly consumed raw tomatoes reduced the risk of prostate cancer by 11%, while men who regularly consumed cooked tomatoes reduced the risk of prostate cancer by 19%.

In brief, tomato intake has been shown to lower blood pressure in cardiovascular disease patients and reduce the risk of prostate cancer. The meta-analytical results evince that tomatoes may alleviate inflammation in the heart and vascular system, inhibit the growth and proliferation of prostate cancer cells, and prevent the incidence of prostate cancer. It is recommended that tomatoes should be included in a nutrient-balanced diet to prevent and treat chronic diseases, particularly cardiovascular disease and prostate cancer.

Table 27.1. Meta-analytical Confirmation of Tomato Intake Associated with Lower Risks of Cardiovascular Disease and Prostate Cancer

Chronic Disease	Risk Reduction, Tomatoes
Cardiovascular disease	Cardiovascular disease patients who regularly consumed tomatoes decreased systolic pressure by 5.7 mmHg.
Prostate cancer	Men who regularly consumed raw tomatoes and cooked tomatoes reduced the risk of prostate cancer by 11% and 19%, respectively. Daily intake of 9–21 mg of lycopene supplement reduced the risk of prostate cancer by 21%.

• Recommendation

Prevention — For people at risk of chronic diseases: men should consume ½ cup of chopped tomato, twice per day and three times per week, and women should consume ½ cup of chopped tomato, twice per day and three times per week.

Treatment — For chronic disease patients: men should consume ½ cup of chopped tomato, twice per day and five times per week, and women should consume ½ cup of chopped tomato, twice per day and four times per week.

Material: Raw tomato contains a higher amount of Vitamin C, while cooked tomato contains a higher amount of lycopene. Alternate eating raw and cooked tomato. One cup of chopped raw tomato is about 200 grams, while one cup of chopped cooked tomato is about 240 grams.

28

Vegetables

How are vegetables classified?

Depending on the season of the year, more than 100 different kinds of vegetables can be found in the grocery stores in the United States. Vegetables can be divided into five types according to their major nutrient contents: green leafy vegetables (kale, spinach, Swiss beet, and lettuce), cruciferous vegetables (cabbage, broccoli, and cauliflower), legumes (black beans, green beans, lentils, lima beans, and soybeans), root vegetables (radish, garlic, ginger, onions, and carrots), and starchy vegetables (potatoes, yams, sweet potatoes, corn, and taro).

Before developing agriculture, humans led a hunting-and-gathering nomadic lifestyle. Any fruits, nuts, plants with edible stems, leaf and roots, and dead or live animals were all fair hunting and gathering targets. In the Neolithic Era, humans started domesticating plants, fruits, and vegetables, and human civilization entered the Agriculture Era. It is rather perplexing that although humans lived in different parts of the world (namely, Mediterranean, Asia, Africa, Europe, and South America), they all coincidentally domesticated plants, fruits, and vegetables, and entered the Agriculture Era about 10,000 years ago.

What are the major nutrients in vegetables?

Vegetables containing no cholesterol are low-fat and low-energy density foods. The major nutrients in vegetables are Vitamin A, Vitamin C, dietary fiber, and essential elements, such as potassium

Table 28.1. Major Nutrient Contents of 19 Different Types of Vegetables

Vegetables	Amount, consumed, g	Sodium, mg	Potassium, mg	Dietary fiber, g	Vitamin A, % DV	Vitamin C, %DV
Asparagus	93	0	230	2	10	15
Persimmon pepper	148	40	220	2	4	190
Broccoli	148	80	460	3	6	220
Carrot	78	60	250	2	110	10
Cauliflower	99	30	270	2	0	100
Celery	110	115	260	2	10	15
Cucumber	99	0	140	1	4	10
Green bean	83	0	200	3	4	10
Cabbage	84	20	190	2	0	70
Scallion	25	10	70	1	2	8
Lettuce	89	10	125	1	6	6
Mushroom	84	15	300	1	0	2
Onion	148	5	190	3	0	20
Potato	148	0	620	2	0	45
Radish	85	55	190	1	0	30
Squash	98	0	260	2	6	30
Corn	90	0	250	2	2	10
Sweet Potato	130	70	440	4	120	30
Tomato	148	20	340	1	20	40

Data adapted from the United States FDA sources; %DV, % daily value based on daily consumption of 2,000 calories.

and sodium. As shown in Table 28.1, carrots and sweet potatoes are excellent sources of Vitamin A, and persimmon pepper, broccoli, and cauliflower are great sources of Vitamin C. All vegetables contain abundant amounts of potassium. Celery has the highest sodium content.

What are the benefits of consuming vegetables?

Vegetable intake is associated with a myriad of health benefits. Vegetables are high in dietary fiber, which augments the feeling of satiety, improves bowel movement, reduces the risk of chronic diseases, and prevents premature mortality. Vegetables are excellent sources of potassium, which can help control blood pressure, regular the acid-alkaline balance, and enhance glucose and insulin metabolism. Antioxidant Vitamin A, Vitamin C, and glutathione in vegetables can strengthen immune defense and help maintain healthy skin and hair. In addition, vegetables contain concentrated amounts of phytochemicals, including carotenoids, lycopene, indoles, isothiocyanates, isoflavones, sulforaphane, phytosterols, zeaxanthin, and lutein. These phytochemicals exhibit anti-cancer properties through a range of mechanisms, including quenching reactive oxygen radicals, supporting detox enzymes and removing carcinogenic compounds in the body, modulating antioxidant enzymes, inhibiting cell proliferation, enhancing cell differentiation, and preventing tumorigenesis.

What Types of Chronic Disease can be Prevented by Consuming Vegetables?

• Meta-analysis

Breast cancer — Women who habitually consume vegetables have lower risk of breast cancer.

Twenty-four research articles investigated the association between vegetable consumption and breast cancer in 15,631 women found that consumption of vegetables reduced the risk of breast cancer by 23%.

Colorectal cancer — Vegetable consumption discernibly lowers the risk of colorectal cancer.

A meta-analysis of eight prospective studies examined the association between vegetable consumption and colorectal cancer including 2,910 colorectal cancer cases showed that consumption of vegetables reduced the risk of colorectal cancer by 14%.

Endometrial cancer — Women who consume 1½ cups of vegetables daily have lower risk of endometrial cancer.

Seventeen research papers examined the relationship between vegetable consumption and endometrial cancer revealed that consumption of vegetables reduced the risk of endometrial cancer by 21%. The dose-response studies revealed that daily consumption of 100 g of vegetables reduced the risk of endometrial cancer by 10%.

Esophageal adenocarcinoma — Frequent consumption of vegetables can diminish the risk of esophageal adenocarcinoma.

A meta-analysis of twelve research articles evaluated the relationship between vegetable consumption and esophageal adenocarcinoma found that vegetable consumption reduced the risk of esophageal adenocarcinoma by 24%.

Esophageal cancer — Vegetable consumption can lessen the risk of esophageal cancer.

Another meta-analysis of thirty-two clinical trials studied the association between vegetable consumption and esophageal cancer including 10,037 esophageal cancer cases revealed that frequent consumption of vegetables reduced the risk of esophageal cancer by 44%.

Hypertension — Regular consumption of vegetables can bring down the risk of hypertension.

A meta-analysis of nine prospective studies investigated the relationship between vegetable consumption and hypertension in 185,676 subjects found that consumption of vegetables reduced the risk of hypertension by 12% in normotensive individuals. The dose-response data revealed that each additional serving of vegetables per day decreased the risk of hypertension by 1.2% in normotensive individuals.

Liver cancer — Consumption of vegetables (1½ cups daily) can noticeably lower the risk of liver cancer.

Nineteen prospective studies investigated the relationship between vegetable consumption and liver cancer in a total of 1,290,045 participants, of which 3,912 were liver cancer cases. The meta-analytical results showed that vegetable consumption reduced the risk of liver cancer by 28%. The dose-response result revealed that each additional intake of 100 g of vegetables per day reduced the risk of liver cancer by 8%.

Lung cancer — Vegetable consumption (1½ cups daily) can lessen the risk of lung cancer.

Seventy-two prospective studies examined the association between vegetable intake and lung cancer in 36,678 people found that consumption of vegetables reduced the risk of lung cancer by 8%. The dose-response analysis revealed that each additional intake of 100 g of vegetables per day reduced the risk of lung cancer by 6%.

Oral cancer — Consumption of vegetables (one cup daily) significantly reduces the risk of oral cancer.

A meta-analysis of sixteen research papers evaluated the relationship between vegetable consumption and oral cancer reported that each additional serving of vegetables per day reduced the risk of oral cancer by 50%.

Pancreatic cancer — People who regularly consume vegetables have lower risk of pancreatic cancer.

Eleven prospective studies examined the association between vegetable consumption and pancreatic cancer showed that consumption of vegetables reduced the risk of pancreatic cancer by 38%.

Premature mortality — Daily consumption of vegetables (1½ cups) reduces the risk of premature death.

Seventy-one prospective studies investigated the relationship between vegetable consumption and premature mortality including 241,000 mortality cases revealed that consumption of vegetables reduced the risk of premature mortality by 7%. In addition, each additional intake of 100 g of vegetables daily reduced the risk of premature mortality by 4%.

Stroke — Consumption of three cups of vegetables daily significantly reduces the incidence of stroke.

A meta-analysis of twelve research articles examined the association between vegetable intake and stroke in 760,629 people including 16,981 stroke cases showed that each additional daily intake of 200 g of vegetables reduced the risk of stroke by 11%.

Type 2 diabetes — Frequent consumption of vegetables, especially dark green leafy vegetables, white vegetables, and cruciferous vegetables, significantly brings down the risk of type 2 diabetes.

Ten prospective studies investigated the relationship between vegetable consumption and type 2 diabetes revealed that each additional serving of vegetables daily reduced the risk of type 2 diabetes by 10%. In addition, each additional one-fifth serving of dark green leafy vegetables daily reduced the risk of type 2 diabetes by 13%. Daily consumption of vegetables, particularly dark green leafy vegetables, could lower the risk of type 2 diabetes. Another meta-analysis of twenty-three research articles examined the association between vegetable intake and type 2 diabetes found that among all vegetables, dark green leafy vegetables, white vegetables and cruciferous vegetables reduced the risk of type 2 diabetes by 23%, 38%, and 28%, respectively.

• Conclusion

Table 28.2 illustrates that consuming vegetables reduced the risk of many chronic diseases, including hypertension, type 2 diabetes, lung cancer, oral cancer, stroke, breast cancer, endometrial cancer, esophageal cancer, pancreatic cancer, colorectal cancer, and premature mortality. Specifically, consumption of vegetables reduced the risk of type 2 diabetes, stroke, and hypertension by 10%, 11%, and 12%, respectively. In addition, consuming vegetables reduced the risk of oral cancer, esophageal cancer, liver cancer, and pancreatic cancer by 50%, 44%, 28%, and 38%, respectively. Moreover, vegetable consumption reduced the risk of endometrial cancer, breast

Table 28.2.   Meta-analytical Confirmation of Vegetable Intake Associated with Lower Risks of 11 Chronic Diseases and Premature Mortality

Chronic Diseases	Reduced Risk, Vegetables
Breast cancer	Vegetables reduced the risk of breast cancer by 23%.
Colorectal cancer	Vegetables reduced the risk of colorectal cancer by 14%.
Endometrial cancer	Vegetables reduced the risk of endometrial cancer by 21%. Women who consumed 100 g of vegetables per day reduced the risk of endometrial cancer by 10%.
Esophageal cancer	Vegetables reduced the risk of esophageal cancer by 44%.
Hypertension	Vegetables reduced the risk of hypertension by 12%. Each additional serving of vegetables per day reduced the risk of hypertension by 1.2%.
Liver cancer	Vegetables reduced the risk of liver cancer by 28%. Each additional intake of 100 g of vegetables per day reduced the risk of liver cancer by 8%.
Lung cancer	Vegetables reduced the risk of lung cancer by 8%. Each additional intake of 100 g of vegetables per day reduced the risk of lung cancer by 6%.
Oral cancer	Vegetables reduced the risk of oral cancer by 50%.
Pancreatic cancer	Vegetables reduced the risk of pancreatic cancer by 38%.
Premature mortality	Vegetables reduced the risk of all-cause mortality by 7%. Each additional intake of 100 g of vegetables reduced the risk of all-cause mortality by 4%.
Stroke	Daily intake of 200 g of vegetables reduced the risk of stroke by 11%.
Type 2 diabetes	Vegetables reduced the risk of type 2 diabetes by 10%. Consumption of dark green leafy vegetables and white vegetables reduced the risk of type 2 diabetes by 23% and 38%, respectively.

cancer, and colorectal cancer by 21%, 23%, and 14%, respectively. In other words, vegetable intake is associated with lower risks of gastrointestinal cancers and gynecological cancers. Furthermore, vegetables reduced the risk of lung cancer by 8% and the risk of premature mortality by 7%.

In conclusion, vegetable intake can lower the risk of hypertension, type 2 diabetes, and stroke, as well as the risk of many types of cancers, including oral cancer, esophageal cancer, lung cancer, liver cancer, pancreatic cancer, colorectal cancer, breast cancer, and premature mortality. Adding vegetables to a healthy diet can prevent many chronic diseases and promote longevity.

• Recommendation

Prevention — For people at risk of chronic diseases: men should consume ½ cup of cooked vegetables twice per day, and women should consume ⅓ cup of cooked vegetables twice per day.

Treatment — For chronic disease patients: men should consume ½ cup of cooked vegetables three times per day, and women should consume ⅓ cup of cooked vegetables three times per day.

Materials: There is a wide selection of vegetables, such as asparagus, persimmon pepper, kale, spinach, Swiss chide, celery, cucumber, cabbage, scallion, mushroom, onion, and the like. Every day select five different color in-season vegetables. One cup of cooked vegetables is about 237 grams in weight.

29

Vegetables and Fruits

We have already talked about how fruit intake or vegetable intake alone in prevention of chronic diseases. People who love fruits often consume vegetables as well.

What Types of Chronic Disease can be Prevented by Consuming Vegetables and Fruits?

• Meta-analysis

Breast cancer — Women who regularly consume fruits and vegetables have lower risk of breast cancer.

A meta-analysis of 12 research articles studied the relationship between consumption of fruits and vegetables and breast cancer in 181,906 women including 9,513 breast cancer cases. The results showed that consumption of fruits and vegetables rich in flavonoids (e.g., citrus fruits, berries, apples, legumes, soy foods, and radishes) reduced the risk of breast cancer by 12%, and consumption of fruits and vegetables rich in flavonols (e.g., blueberries, apples, onions, kale, leeks, and broccoli) reduced the risk of breast cancer by 17%.

Cardiovascular disease — Daily consumption of ten cups of fruits and vegetables can discernibly reduce the risk of cardiovascular disease.

Ninety-five prospective studies examined the association between fruit and vegetable intake and cardiovascular disease found that a daily consumption of 200 g of fruits and vegetables reduced the risk of cardiovascular disease by 8%. The results denote that daily intake of three cups of fruits and vegetables can diminish the risk of cardiovascular disease. Another meta-analysis of 47 prospective studies evaluated the relationship between fruit and vegetable consumption and cardiovascular disease in 1,498,909 people including 44,013 cardiovascular disease cases. The results showed that a daily intake of 800 g of fruits and vegetables reduced the risk of cardiovascular disease by 17%.

Cognitive impairment — Elderly people who consumed 1½ cups of fruits and vegetables daily have lower risk of cognitive impairment.

A meta-analysis of five prospective studies examined the association between fruit and vegetable consumption and cognitive impairment in 31,104 people including 4,583 cognitive impairment and dementia cases found that the consumption of fruits and vegetables reduced the risk of cognitive impairment and dementia by 20%. The dose-response analysis revealed that each additional intake of 100 g of fruits and vegetables per day reduced the risk of cognitive impairment and dementia by 13%.

Colorectal cancer — Regular consumption of fruits and vegetables can lessen the risk of colorectal cancer.

Twenty-two prospective studies investigated the relationship between fruit and vegetable consumption and colorectal cancer revealed that consumption of fruits and vegetables reduced the risk of colorectal cancer by 18%.

Esophageal adenocarcinoma — Regular consumption of fruits and vegetables can curtail the risk of esophageal adenocarcinoma.

Twelve clinical trial reports evaluated the association between fruit and vegetable consumption and esophageal adenocarcinoma revealed that consumption of fruits and vegetables reduced 32% risk of esophageal adenocarcinoma.

Hypertension — People who frequently consume fruits and vegetables have lower risk of hypertension.

Nine prospective studies examined the relationship between fruit and vegetable consumption and hypertension in 185,676 people reported that consumption of fruits and vegetables reduced the risk of hypertension by 10% in normotensive individuals.

Oral cancer — Frequent consumption of fruits and vegetables can greatly reduce the risk of oral cancer.

Ten case-control studies investigated the association between fruit and vegetable consumption and oral cancer including 5,959 head and neck cancer cases, and 12,248 control subjects. The results showed that consumption of fruits and vegetables reduced the risk of oral cancer by 46%.

Premature mortality — People who habitually consume fruits and vegetables have lower risk of premature mortality, including disease-specific and all-cause mortalities.

Seventy-five prospective studies examined the association between fruit and vegetable consumption and premature mortality found that a daily intake of 200 g of fruits and vegetables reduced coronary heart disease mortality, stroke mortality, cardiovascular disease mortality, cancer mortality, and all-cause mortality by 8%, 16%, 8%, 3%, and 10%, respectively. In addition, a daily consumption of 800 g of fruits and vegetables was found to provide the most protective effect against premature mortalities, including all-cause mortality and disease-specific mortalities. Another meta-analysis of ten prospective studies investigated the relationship between fruit and vegetable consumption and premature mortality including 31,210 breast cancer mortality cases revealed that breast cancer patients who consumed more fruits and vegetables had an 8% lower risk of breast cancer mortality compare to breast cancer patients who consumed less fruits and vegetables.

Stomach cancer — Regular consumption of fruits and vegetables can bring down the risk of stomach cancer.

A meta-analysis of four prospective studies on dietary habits of 191,232 Japanese, including 2,995 stomach cancer cases, found that consumption of fruits and vegetables reduced the risk of stomach cancer in men and women by 11% and 17%, respectively.

Stroke — High consumption of fruits and vegetables decreases the risk of stroke.

Twelve prospective studies investigated the relationship between fruit and vegetable intake and stroke in 760,629 people including 16,981 stroke cases revealed that regular consumption of fruits and vegetables reduced the risk of stroke by 21%. In brief, people who consumed fruits and vegetables had lower incidence of stroke. Another meta-analysis of eight prospective studies examined the association between fruit and vegetable intake and stroke in 257,551 people including 4,917 stroke cases showed that a daily consumption of 3 servings of fruits and vegetables reduced the risk of stroke by 11% and a daily consumption of 3 to 5 servings of fruits and vegetables reduced the risk of stroke by 26%.

• Conclusion

The meta-analytical data presented in Table 29.1 illustrates that consumption of fruits and vegetables reduced the risk of chronic diseases, including type 2 diabetes, cardiovascular disease, stroke, oral cancer, esophageal adenocarcinoma, stomach cancer, breast cancer, endometrial cancer, colorectal cancer, cognitive impairment, and the risk of premature mortality. Consumption of fruits and vegetables reduced the risk of hypertension and stroke by 10% and 21%, respectively. In addition, consumption of fruits and vegetables reduced the risk of oral cancer, esophageal adenocarcinoma, and colorectal cancer by 46%, 32%, and 18%, respectively. For women, consumption of fruits and vegetables reduced the risk of breast cancer by 12–17%. Moreover, consumption of fruits and vegetables reduced the risk of cognitive impairment by 20% in elderly people. Finally, consumption of fruits and vegetables reduced the risk of coronary disease mortality by 8% and the risk of stroke mortality by 16%.

Table 29.1. Meta-analytical Confirmation of Fruit and Vegetable Consumption Associated with Lower Risks of Chronic Diseases and Premature Mortality

Chronic Diseases	Reduced Risk, Fruits and Vegetables
Breast cancer	Fruits and vegetables rich in flavonoids reduced the risk of breast cancer by 12%. Fruits and vegetables rich in flavones reduced the risk of breast cancer by 17%.
Cardiovascular disease	Daily intake of 200 g of fruits and vegetables reduced the risk of cardiovascular disease by 8%. Daily intake of 800 g of fruits and vegetables reduced the risk of cardiovascular disease by 17%.
Colorectal cancer	Fruits and vegetables reduced the risk of colorectal cancer by 18%.
Esophageal adenocarcinoma	Fruits and vegetables reduced the risk of esophageal adenocarcinoma by 32%.
Hypertension	Fruits and vegetables reduced the risk of hypertension by 10%.
Oral cancer	Fruits and vegetables reduced the risk of oral cancer by 46%.
Premature mortality	Daily intake of 200 g of fruits and vegetables reduced the risk of coronary heart disease mortality, stroke mortality, cardiovascular disease mortality, cancer mortality, and all-cause mortality by 8%, 16%, 8%, 3%, and 10%, respectively. Fruits and vegetables reduced the risk of breast cancer mortality by 8%.
Stomach cancer	Fruits and vegetables reduced the risk of stomach cancer in men and women by 11% and 17%, respectively.
Stroke	Fruits and vegetables reduced the risk of stroke by 21%. Daily intake of 3 servings and 3–5 servings of fruits and vegetables reduced the risk of stroke by 11% and 26%, respectively.

In conclusion, the intake of fruits and vegetables is associated with lower risks of cardiovascular diseases, stroke, and premature mortality. Frequent consumption of fruits and vegetables curtailed the risk of oral cancer, esophageal adenocarcinoma, and colorectal cancer. For women, fruit and vegetable consumption lessened the risk of breast cancer. For elderly people, fruit and vegetable consumption reduced the risk of cognitive impairment. It is recommended that fruits and vegetables should be considered excellent food remedies in the prevention and management of chronic diseases including cancers.

• Recommendation

Prevention — For people at risk of chronic disease: men should consume ½ cup of cooked vegetables, twice per day and ½ cup of chopped fresh fruits, twice per day, and women should consume ⅓ cup of cooked vegetables, twice per day, and ½ cup of chopped fresh fruits, twice per day.

Treatment — For chronic disease patients: men should consume ½ cup of cooked vegetables, three times per day and ½ cup of chopped fresh fruits, three times per day, and women should consume ⅓ cup of cooked vegetables, three times per day and ½ cup of chopped fresh fruits, three times per day.

Materials: Select daily five different colored vegetables and five different fruits. One cup of cooked green leafy vegetables is about 237 g and one cup of chopped fresh fruits is about 175 g.

30

Whole Grains

What are whole grains?

In their natural state, whole grains, such as wheat, brown rice, oats, barley, quinoa, rye, sorghum, and buckwheat, are comprised of bran, germ, and endosperm. The outer layer of a whole grain is the bran, which is rich in dietary fiber, B vitamins, essential elements, and phytochemicals. The germ contains high amounts of proteins, lipids, and essential elements, and under favorable conditions, it can germinate to become a small plant. The endosperm holds bulk quantities of carbohydrates and lipids, which are used as fuels to support the growth of the germ during germination and growth phases.

In contrast, a refined grain is an imperfect grain, which lacks either the bran, germ, or endosperm. White rice and white flour are refined grains, which have only the endosperm, not the bran or germ.

Compared to refined grains, whole grains are more susceptible to mold and are harder to store. By the late 18th century, the invention of the grain milling machinery allowed the industrial-scale production of refined grains, mainly, white rice and white flour. These tasty refined grains were easy to produce and store, and quickly became popular staple foods in the world. Unfortunately, long-term consumption of white rice and white flour caused Vitamin B1-deficient Beriberi disease and Vitamin B3-deficient Pellagra disease; both diseases were prevalent worldwide in the

19th century. To circumvent these health problems, white rice and white flour are now fortified with Vitamin B1, Vitamin B2, Vitamin B3, folic acid, and iron in most countries. Nevertheless, fortified refined grains are still not nutritionally equivalent to whole grains. A healthy diet that includes whole grains, such as brown rice and whole wheat, can resolve those nutrient-deficient problems associated with the refined grains.

The history of whole grains can be traced all the way back to the early human civilization. Below is a brief history of three types of whole grains.

Wheat — Wheat was a staple food for hunter-gatherer humans. In the Paleolithic Age, wild wheat was abundant. During the growing season, a hunter-gatherer could readily collect a sizable amount of wild wheat from the field to feed his whole family. In the Neolithic Age, farmers in Iraq, Iran, and Palestine started domesticating wild wheat. In addition to eating wheat grains, they unknowingly utilized yeast that naturally adhered to wild wheat grains to bake bread and brew beer. Around 2000 BCE, people in China began cultivating wild wheat. Perhaps owing to differences in wild wheat species, domesticating wild wheat in China did not lead to bread and beer; instead, the Chinese people created noodles and unique noodle cultures.

Corn — Seven thousand years ago, people living in Central Mexico took a wild grass called teosinte and domesticated it to become corn. Corn cultivation later spread to Ecuador, but according to archeological relics, it did not reach North America until the 1st century when the Pueblo people grew corn crops. In the late 15th century, Christopher Columbus and his fleets reached the New World and brought corn seeds back to Europe. Corn became a staple food in Spain, Italy, and other Southern European countries in the subsequent centuries. Since the late 19th century, the United States has been the largest corn producing country in the world; however, most of the corn grown in the United States has been used in animal agriculture as cattle and chicken feeds.

Oats — Like wheat and barley, oats are best grown in temperate regions. In the Neolithic Age, humans began domesticating wild wheat and wild barley, but showed little interest in wild oats, because humans regarded them as wild grass. In the Bronze Age, domesticated oats, which thrive in cold and wet environments, appeared in Europe. In the 17th century, horse wagons became a popular means of public transportation in North America so oats were grown as horse feed, mainly by Irish immigrants. By the late 19th century, automobiles replaced horse wagons as the primary means of public transportation, thus ending an era of horse wagon and the need of oat grains as horse feed. Oat production drastically declined until the 1920s when oatmeal gained popularity as a favorite American breakfast.

What are the major nutrients in whole grains?

The major nutrients in whole grains are carbohydrates, proteins, lipids, dietary fiber, B vitamins, and essential elements. Table 30.1 illustrates

Table 30.1.   Major Nutrient Contents of 6 Common Whole Grains

	Wheat	Brown Rice	Quinoa	Oats	Rye	Millet	Unit
Protein	5.67	3.39	6.35	7.60	4.65	4.96	g
Lipid	0.69	1.44	2.73	3.11	0.73	1.90	g
Carbohydrate	32.03	31.31	28.87	29.82	34.14	32.78	g
Dietary fiber	5.5	1.6	3.1	4.8	6.8	3.8	g
Calcium	13	4	21	24	11	4	mg
Iron	1.44	0.58	2.06	2.12	1.18	1.35	mg
Magnesium	57	52	89	80	50	51	mg
Phosphate	130	140	206	235	149	128	mg
Potassium	163	112	253	193	230	88	mg
Sodium	1	2	2	1	1	2	mg
Zinc	1.19	0.96	1.40	1.79	1.19	0.76	mg
Copper	0.20	0.13	0.27	0.28	0.17	0.34	mg
Manganese	1.79	1.68	0.92	2.21	1.16	0.73	mg

Table 30.1. (*Continued*)

	Wheat	Brown Rice	Quinoa	Oats	Rye	Millet	Unit
Selenium	31.8	10.5	3.8	—	6.3	1.2	µg
Vitamin C	0	0	0	0	0	0	mg
Vitamin B1	0.17	0.24	0.16	0.34	0.14	0.19	mg
Vitamin B2	0.05	0.04	0.14	0.06	0.11	0.13	mg
Vitamin B3	2.46	2.92	0.68	0.43	1.92	2.12	mg
Vitamin B5	0.43	0.67	0.35	0.61	0.66	0.38	mg
Vitamin B6	0.14	0.22	0.22	0.05	0.13	0.17	mg
Vitamin B9	17	10	83	25	17	38	µg

All data is calculated based on 45 grams of dried whole grains and is adapted from the USDA.
unit: g — grams and mg — milligrams.

the major nutrient contents of six common whole grains, among which oats has the highest protein content and rye has the highest dietary fiber content. It is worth noting that all whole grains are excellent sources of essential elements, such as calcium, phosphate, and potassium, and essential trace elements, such as iron, zinc, copper, manganese, and selenium, as well as B vitamins, including Vitamin B1, Vitamin B2, Vitamin B3, Vitamin B5, Vitamin B6, and Vitamin B9.

What are the health benefits of whole grains?

Whole grains are rich in dietary fiber, which can lower postprandial glucose responses and insulin demand. High blood insulin level can promote appetite and stimulate lipid storage in the adipose tissues and increase the risk of obesity. Dietary fiber can also help regulate lipid and glucose metabolism in the liver, increase bile acid excretion from the gallbladder, lower blood cholesterol level, and reduce the risk of hypercholesterolemia. As aforementioned, in the digestive tract, through bacterial fermentation, dietary fibers can release short chain fatty acids that exert antioxidant activities to protect against oxidative damage in the digestive tract as well as in the rest of the body.

In addition, whole grains are excellent sources of B vitamins such as pantothenic acid, thiamin, niacin, riboflavin, and folate, all of which have been shown to reduce the risk of cancer. Furthermore, whole grains are rich in phenolic acids, phytoestrogens, and lignans, phytochemicals that can modulate the hormonal balance and protect against carcinogenesis.

The United States Food and Drug Administration (FDA) allows food items that contain more than 51% of whole grains to include a label claiming, "diets rich in whole grain foods and other plant foods and low in total fat, saturated fat and cholesterol may reduce the risk of heart disease and some cancers."

What Types of Chronic Disease can be Prevented by Consuming Whole Grains?

• Meta-analysis

Cardiovascular disease — Daily consumption of whole grains (two ounces) can greatly lower the risk of cardiovascular disease.

An umbrella meta-analysis review of 21 published meta-analytic papers investigated the relationship between whole grain consumption and cardiovascular disease. The results found that a daily intake of 45 g of whole grains reduced the risk of cardiovascular disease by 29%.

Colorectal cancer — Daily consumption of whole grains (four ounces) noticeably decreases the risk of colorectal cancer.

One hundred and eleven prospective studies examined the association between whole grain consumption and colorectal cancer revealed that a daily consumption of 90 g of whole grains reduced the risk of colorectal cancer by 17%.

Hypercholesterolemia — Regular consumption of whole grains reduces blood cholesterol levels and favorably influences blood lipid profiles in patients with hypercholesterolemia.

Forty-five prospective studies and 21 double-blind randomized clinical trials investigated the relationship between whole grain consumption and hypercholesterolemia. The results indicated that whole grain consumption decreased total cholesterol by

15.1 mg/dL and LDL cholesterol by 13.1 mg/dL in hypercholesterolemic patients.

Pancreatic cancer — Consumption of whole grains diminishes the risk of pancreatic cancer, particularly in Americans.

A meta-analysis of eight research papers examined the association between whole grain consumption and pancreatic cancer including 2,500 pancreatic cancer cases found that consumption of whole grain reduced the risk of pancreatic cancer by 24%. Further analysis revealed that whole grains reduced the risk of pancreatic cancer in Americans and Europeans by 36% and 5%, respectively.

Premature mortality — A daily consumption of whole grains (four ounces) can profoundly bring down the risk of premature mortality.

A meta-analysis of ten prospective studies investigated the relationship between whole grain consumption and premature mortality in 782,751 subjects, of which 92,647 are mortality cases. The results showed that a daily intake of 30 g of whole grain reduced the risk of all-cause mortality, cardiovascular mortality, and coronary heart disease mortality by 7%, 5%, and 8%, respectively. A daily consumption of one ounce of whole grains can significantly decrease the risk of premature mortality. Another meta-analysis of twenty prospective studies investigated the association of whole grain consumption and premature mortality including 104,061 all-cause mortality cases, 26,352 cardiovascular disease mortality cases, and 34,797 cancer mortality cases 104,061. The results revealed that a daily consumption of 50 g of whole grain reduced the risk of all-cause, cardiovascular, myocardial infarction, and cancer mortalities by 22%, 30%, 32%, and 18%, respectively. In brief, daily consumption of two ounces of whole grains could discernibly lower the risk of premature mortality. Further supporting evidence about the benefits of whole grains is presented in a meta-analysis of forty-five prospective studies including 100,726 all-cause mortality cases showed that daily consumption of 90 g of whole grains reduced the risk of all-cause mortality, diabetes mortality, and infectious disease mortalities by 17%, 51%, and 26%, as well as reduced the risk of cancer and respiratory disease mortalities by 15% and 22%, respectively.

Stroke — Whole grain consumption significantly curtails the risk of stroke.

Six prospective studies explored the association between whole grain intake and risk of stroke found that whole grain consumption lessened the risk of stroke in men and women by 14% and 22%, respectively. The dose response results revealed that daily intake of 90 g of whole grains reduced the risk of stroke by 12%.

Type 2 diabetes — A daily consumption of whole grain (three servings; 15 g each serving) can significantly lower the risk of type 2 diabetes.

Eight prospective studies evaluated the relationship between whole grain consumption and type 2 diabetes in a total of 316,051 participants, of which 15,573 were type 2 diabetes cases. The meta-analytical results showed that consumption of three servings (15 g each serving) of whole grains daily reduced the risk of type 2 diabetes by 20%.

• Conclusion

The meta-analytical results confirm that consuming whole grains reduced total cholesterol and LDL cholesterol levels in hypercholesterolemic patients. In addition, whole grains reduced the risk of cardiovascular disease, type 2 diabetes, and colorectal cancer by 29%, 20%, and 17%, respectively (see Table 30.2). Whole grain consumption is also found to lower the risk of stroke in men and women by 14% and 22%, respectively. Furthermore, whole grains reduced the risk of premature mortality, including the risk of diabetes mortality, myocardial infarction mortality, and cardiovascular disease mortality by 51%, 32%, and 30%, respectively.

In conclusion, whole grains are excellent food remedies to prevent and treat hypercholesterolemia, type 2 diabetes, cardiovascular disease, colorectal cancer, and premature mortality and should be included as part of a healthy diet to prevent and treat chronic diseases.

Table 30.2. Meta-analytical Confirmation of Whole Grain Intake Associated with Lower Risks of Chronic Diseases and Premature Mortality

Chronic Diseases	Reduced Risk, Whole Grains
Cardiovascular disease	Daily intake of 45 g of whole grains reduced the risk of cardiovascular disease by 29%.
Colorectal cancer	Daily intake of 90 g of whole grains reduced the risk of colorectal cancer by 17%.
Hypercholesterolemia	Whole grains reduced total cholesterol level by 15.1 mg/dL and LDL cholesterol level by 13.1 mg/dL in patients with hypercholesterolemia.
Pancreatic cancer	Whole grains reduced the risk of pancreatic cancer by 24%.
Premature mortality	Daily consumption of 30 g of whole grains reduced the risk of all-cause mortality, cardiovascular disease mortality, coronary heart disease mortality by 7%, 5%, and 8%, respectively.
	Daily consumption of 50 g of whole grains reduced all-cause mortality, cardiovascular mortality, myocardial mortality, and cancer mortality by 22%, 30%, 32%, and 18%, respectively.
	Daily consumption of 90 g of whole grains reduced the risk of all-cause mortality, cancer mortality, respiratory disease mortality, diabetes mortality, and infectious disease mortality by 17%, 15%, 22%, 51%, 26%, respectively.
Stroke	Whole grain consumption reduced the risk of stroke in men and women by 14% and 22%, respectively.
	Daily intake of 90 g of whole grains reduced the risk of stroke by 12%.
Type 2 diabetes	Daily consumption of three servings (15 g each serving) of whole grains reduced the risk of type 2 diabetes by 20%.

• Recommendation

Prevention — For people at risk of chronic disease: men should consume ½ cup of cooked whole grain twice per day or two slices of whole wheat bread twice per day and, women should consume ¼ cup of cooked whole grain twice per day or one slice of whole wheat bread thrice a day.

Treatment — For chronic disease patients: men should consume ½ cup of cooked whole grain thrice per day or two slices of whole wheat bread thrice a day, and women should consume ½ cup of cooked whole grain twice per day or one slice of whole wheat bread thrice a day.

Materials: Whole grains include wheat, brown rice, oats, rye, and millet. One cup of cooked brown rice is about 195–200 g, and one slice of whole wheat bread is about 42.5 g.

Part Two

Seven Disease-causative Foods

The human body is made up of 1.32 trillion cells and whether you are awake or sleeping, each of these cells in your body dutifully performs and fulfills its specific role and responsibility. Each cell is comprised of hundreds of thousands of molecules, and each molecule has its designated role and significance within the cell. Like a busy factory, all molecules in a cell are not static; they are constantly moving or rotating. Some molecules carry out repair-and-rebuild work, and others are responsible for producing energy or transporting materials into or out of the cell. All molecules in a cell must work in an organized and cooperative manner for the cell to perform its specific role and responsibility, for example, stomach cells to make stomach acid and pancreatic cells to produce insulin. To do that, every cell needs raw materials such as nutrients, vitamins, and essential elements. In Part One, we talked about thirty clinically proven food remedies that can provide necessary nutrients, vitamins, and essential elements to all the cells in the body and allow them to perform their specific roles and responsibilities.

Researchers have also employed the meta-analysis method to study the dietary habits of millions of people worldwide and have identified seven disease-causative foods that are linked to chronic diseases and cancers. These harmful food items include red meat, processed meat, sugar-sweetened beverages, artificially-sweetened beverages, high glycemic-load foods, high-salt diet, and eggs.

Consumption of these harmful foods not only cannot provide necessary nutrients, vitamins, and essential elements to the cells, but also can cause injuries to the cells, leading to pathological changes in the structure and function of the cells, and eventually destroying the cells' abilities to perform their specific roles and responsibilities (e.g., stomach cells can no longer make stomach acid or pancreatic cells can no longer produce insulin). Granted, our bodies are equipped with repair-and-rebuild mechanisms, so that occasional injuries to the cells caused by harmful foods may not impose any lasting damage. However, habitual consumption of these harmful foods can overwhelm repair-and-rebuild mechanisms, bring on permanent pathological changes, and lead to chronic diseases. Furthermore, if the DNA in one stomach cell mutates and transforms into a cancerous cell, immune cells in the body will likely kill this lone cancerous cell. However, if you habitually consume red meat and processed meat, which are known to contain carcinogenic compounds, these carcinogenic compounds can hasten the growth and proliferation of that lone cancerous stomach cell to become stomach cancer. Hence, consuming harmful foods can heighten the risk of chronic diseases as well as the risk of cancer.

31

Red Meat

About 10,000 years ago, human societies transformed from the hunters-gatherers to agricultural societies by cultivating whole grains, fruits, and vegetables, and raising cows and sheep. By 8000 BCE, in addition to whole grains, vegetables, and fruits, humans also consumed beef and lamb. However, during that time, red meat was still rare and expensive, and only wealthy people and nobles could afford it; most peasants ate mostly whole grains, vegetables, and fruits. The price of red meat was expensive and cost prohibitive to common people for several thousands of years until the 17th century. In the 17th century, new European immigrants, particularly the British, brought several breeds of cattle and fed them with wild grasses that grew on the vast prairie of North America. The beef industry was born on the American soil in the following enduring centuries. Since then, the price of beef has dropped precipitously. By 1950, the price of beef was even cheaper than the price of chicken in the United States grocery stores. As a result, beef, a high energy-density food, became a favorite meat on the American's dinner table. According to the data from the USDA, beef consumption among Americans is now about 85.5 pounds per capita per year. Undeniably, beef has abundant proteins, lipids, and other nutrients. But humans are not like lions or tigers, and our bodies are not designed to digest and absorb large amounts of meat and fats. The extra meat and fats wreak havoc on our bodies year after year, altering metabolism and hormonal balance, causing systemic and irreparable damage to our health.

Which countries have high beef consumption in the world?

In 2016, global beef consumption was about 130 billion pounds, which is equivalent to every living person on this planet consuming 17.4 pounds of beef per year. Uruguay and Argentina are the top two countries in the world with the highest beef consumption per capita per year as shown in Table 31.1. Every person in those two countries consumed on average more than 120 pounds of beef

Table 31.1.   Twenty Highest Beef Consumption Countries in the World

Countries	Beef Consumption, per Capita per Year (Pound)
Uruguay	136.9
Argentina	123.0
United States	85.5
Brazil	83.3
Paraguay	78.5
Australia	77.8
Canada	65.3
New Zealand	64.4
Kazakhstan	59.1
Hong Kong	52.4
Chile	52.1
Uzbekistan	47.4
Colombia	42.3
Venezuela	40.1
Mexico	40.1
EU-27	36.6
Russia	36.6
South Africa	30.9
South Korea	27.6
Iran	21.6

The data adapted from the USDA 2011.

each year. Beef consumption of the United States ranks the 3rd, right behind Uruguay and Argentina.

Why is beef consumption harmful to health?

- Hemoglobin — Cutting a piece of raw steak, you will notice red-pink juices flowing out of it. The red-pink juices are hemoglobin molecules in the meat reacting with oxygen molecules in the air. Beef contains high amounts of hemoglobin, which gives it the reddish-pink color and the name "red meat". Our bodies need a trace amount of iron but cannot possibly absorb the large amount of iron in red meat. Excessive iron can react with oxygen to generate harmful free radicals, such as hydroxyl radicals. These free radicals cause oxidative damage to proteins, lipids, and nucleic acids in the cells and destroy the cells' normal functions. If your cardiac cells or kidney cells cannot perform their normal functions, you may have an increased risk of heart disease or kidney disease.
- Animal fat — A piece of lean beef contains at least 15% of fats. High fat foods usually taste good. However, our bodies can only digest a small amount of saturated fats. Excessive fats in red meat are transported via the blood circulation and stored in subcutaneous and visceral fat tissues, thus increasing the risk of obesity and metabolic syndrome.
- Carcinogens — Raw red meat generally contains no carcinogen. Yet, when heated to high temperature, red meat can produce heterocyclic amine and polycyclic hydrocarbon carcinogens. Consumption of barbecued beef or charcoal-cooked steak can increase the risk of cancers, including breast cancer, lung cancer, prostate cancer, and colorectal cancer. The International Agency for Research on Cancer, the cancer research agency of World Health Organization, has recommended that red meat be considered as Group 2A human carcinogens.
- L-Carnitine — Beef contains a high amount of L-carnitine, which is a naturally occurring compound that facilitates the transport of fatty acids to the mitochondria and enhances

energy production. However, bacteria living in the gut can transform L-carnitine to trimethylamine-N-oxide. A high blood level of trimethylamine-N-oxide is associated with an increased risk of heart disease, stroke, and even premature death.

What Types of Chronic Disease can be Caused by Red Meat Consumption?

• Meta-analysis

Breast cancer — Women who regularly consume red meat have an elevated risk of breast cancer.

A meta-analysis of twelve prospective studies investigated the association between red meat and breast cancer in a total of 1,154,364 subjects, of which 23,667 were breast cancer cases. The results showed that each additional serving of red meat per day increased the risk of breast cancer by 13%.

Colorectal adenomas — People who consume red meat (four ounces daily) significantly augment the risk of colorectal adenomas.

Twenty-nine prospective studies evaluated the association between red meat and colorectal adenomas found that consumption of beef increased the risk of colorectal adenomas by 11%, and consumption of lamb increased the risk of colorectal adenomas by 24%. The results confirm that high consumption of red meat including beef and lamb heightened the incidence of colorectal adenomas. Another meta-analysis of 26 research articles examined the relationship between red meat and colorectal adenomas revealed that a daily consumption of 100 g of red meat increased the risk of colorectal adenomas by 27%.

Colorectal cancer — Habitual consumption of red meat exacerbates the risk of colorectal cancer.

One hundred and sixteen prospective studies investigated the association between red meat and colorectal cancer found that red meat consumption increased the risk of colorectal cancer by 13%.

Esophageal cancer — High consumption of red meat greatly increases the risk of esophageal cancer.

A meta-analysis of thirty-five research papers evaluated the association between red meat and esophageal cancer showed that consumption of red meat increased the risk of esophageal cancer by 55%.

Heart disease — People who regularly consume red meat have higher risk of heart disease (coronary heart disease and heart failure).

One hundred and twenty-three prospective studies on the relationship between red meat consumption and heart disease found that consumption of red meat increased the risk of coronary heart disease by 15% and the risk of heart failure by 8%.

Lung cancer — Daily consumption of red meat profoundly heightens the incidence of lung cancer.

Thirty-four research articles studied the relationship between red meat and lung cancer revealed that consumption of red meat increased the risk of lung cancer by 44%. The dose-response studies showed that each additional intake of 120 g of red meat per day increased the risk of lung cancer by 35%.

Oral cancer — Red meat consumption can discernibly increase the risk of oral cancer.

A meta-analysis of thirteen research papers examined the association between red meat and oral cancer in a total of 501,730 participants, of which 4,104 were oral cancer cases. The results showed that red meat consumption increased the risk of oral cancer by 5%.

Pancreatic cancer — High consumption of red meat greatly elevates the risk of pancreatic cancer.

Eleven clinical research papers evaluated the relationship between red meat and pancreatic cancer revealed that consumption of red meat increased the risk of pancreatic cancer by 48%.

Premature mortality — Consuming red meat (four ounces daily) can significantly elevate the risk of premature mortality.

Thirteen prospective studies examined the relationship between red meat and premature mortality in 1,674,272 people showed that consumption of red meat increased the risk of cardiovascular disease mortality by 16% and cardiovascular disease by 16%. In addition, each additional intake of 100 g of red meat increased the risk of all-cause mortality by 10%. Analysis confirms that people who consumed four ounces of red meat daily heighten the risk of premature mortality from cardiovascular disease. Another meta-analysis of twelve prospective studies investigated the association between red meat and premature mortality including 321,227 all-cause mortality showed that consumption of red meat increased the risk of all-cause mortality by 10%. In addition, each additional intake of 100 g of red meat per day increased the risk of all-cause mortality by 10%.

Stomach cancer — People who habitually consume red meat have profoundly higher risk of stomach cancer.

Fifty-seven prospective studies evaluated the relationship between red meat and stomach cancer including a total of 2,133,858 participants, of which 20,293 were stomach cancer cases. The meta-analytical results indicated that consumption of red meat increased the risk of stomach cancer by 67%.

Stroke — Daily consumption of red meat (four ounces) exacerbates the incidence of stroke.

Seven prospective studies investigated the relationship between red meat and stroke included 2,079,236 subjects, of which 21,730 were stroke cases found that red meat increased the risk of total stroke by 13%, which confirms that people who regularly consumed red meat augmented the incidence of stroke. Another meta-analysis of five prospective studies evaluated the association between red meat and stroke included 239,251 participants, of which 9,593 were stroke cases found that red meat increased the risk of total stroke by 9% and the risk of ischemic stroke by 13%. In addition, each additional intake of 100 g of red meat per day increased the risk of stroke by 13%.

Type 2 diabetes — Consumption of red meat (four ounces daily) greatly increases the risk of type 2 diabetes.

Fourteen prospective studies examined the relationship between red meat and type 2 diabetes in 50,345 people showed that a daily consumption of 100 g of red meat increased the fasting glucose level by 0.67 mg/dL. In brief, people who consumed four ounces of red meat per day had an elevated fasting glucose level and an increased risk of type 2 diabetes. Another meta-analysis of three prospective studies evaluated the association between red meat and type 2 diabetes including 13,759 type 2 diabetes cases, found that each additional daily serving of red meat daily increased the risk of type 2 diabetes by 14%. The dose-response studies revealed that each additional intake of 100 g of red meat daily increased the risk of type 2 diabetes by 19%.

• Conclusion

Table 31.2 illustrates that consumption of red meat increased the risk of heart failure, ischemic stroke, and type 2 diabetes by 8%, 13% and 14%, respectively. In addition, consuming red meat also increased the risk of esophageal cancer, stomach cancer, pancreatic cancer, and colorectal cancer by 55%, 67%, 48%, and 13%, respectively. For women, red meat increased the risk of breast cancer by 13%. Moreover, consuming red meat increased the risk of all-cause mortality by 10%.

In conclusion, red meat consumption is associated with an increased risk of chronic diseases, including heart failure, stroke, and type 2 diabetes, and gastrointestinal cancers (esophageal cancer, stomach cancer, pancreatic cancer, and colorectal cancer), and breast cancer, as well as an increased risk of premature mortality.

Table 31.2. Meta-analytical Confirmation of Red Meat Consumption Associated with an Increased Risk of Chronic Diseases and Premature Mortality

Chronic Diseases	Increased Risk, Red Meat
Breast cancer	Red meat increased the risk of breast cancer by 13% in both pre- and postmenopausal women.
Colorectal adenomas	Beef and lamb consumption increased the risk of colorectal adenomas by 11% and 24%, respectively. Daily intake of 100 g of red meat increased the risk of colorectal adenomas by 27%.
Colorectal cancer	Red meat increased the risk of colorectal cancer by 13%.
Esophageal cancer	Red meat increased the risk of esophageal cancer by 55%. Daily intake of 120 g of red meat increased the risk of esophageal cancer by 35%.
Heart disease	Red meat increased the risk of coronary heart disease by 15% and heart failure by 8%.
Lung cancer	Red meat increased the risk of lung cancer by 44%. Each additional intake of 120 g of red meat per day increased the risk of lung cancer by 35%.
Oral cancer	Red meat increased the risk of oral cancer by 5%.
Pancreatic cancer	Red meat increased the risk of pancreatic cancer by 48%. Daily consumption of 120 g of red meat increased the risk of pancreatic cancer by 13%.
Premature mortality	Red meat increased the risk of all-cause mortality by 10% and cardiovascular disease mortality by 16%. Daily consumption of 100 g of red meat increased the risk of all-cause mortality by 10%.
Stomach cancer	Red meat increased the risk of stomach cancer by 67%. Beef consumption increased the risk of stomach cancer by 28%.
Stroke	Red meat increased the risk of total stroke and ischemic stroke by 9–13% and 13%, respectively. Daily consumption of 100 g of red meat increased the risk of stroke by 13%.
Type 2 diabetes	Red meat increased the risk of type 2 diabetes by 14%. Daily consumption of 100 g of red meat increased the risk of type 2 diabetes by 19%.

• Recommendation

Prevention — People at risk of chronic disease should not consume more than 4 ounces of red meat per week, and chronic disease patients should avoid consuming any red meat such as beef and lamb.

What Types of Gynecological Cancer can be Caused by Consuming Animal Fats?

• Meta-analysis

Breast cancer — Women who regularly consume animal fats have an increased risk of breast cancer.

Twenty-two prospective studies on the relationship between animal fat consumption and breast cancer in 23,201 women found that high consumption of animal fats increased the risk of breast cancer by 15% in both pre- and postmenopausal women.

Endometrial cancer — Women who frequently consume high amounts of animal fats have greater risks of endometrial cancer.

A meta-analysis of 21 clinical reports investigated the association between animal fat intake and endometrial cancer showed that a daily consumption of 5 g of animal fats increased the risk of endometrial cancer by 5%, and a daily consumption of 10 g of animal fats increased the risk of endometrial cancer by 17% in women on a daily 1,000-calorie diet. The results confirm that women who consumed 5 to 10 g of animal fats per day augmented the risk of endometrial cancer. Another meta-analysis of sixteen research papers examined the relationship between animal fat consumption and endometrial cancer in 563,781 participants, of which 7,556 were endometrial cancer cases. The results revealed that each additional intake of 30 g of animal fats per day increased the risk of endometrial cancer by 17%.

Ovarian cancer — Women who habitually consume animal fats and saturated fats augment incident rates of ovarian cancer.

Eight prospective studies on the association between animal fats and ovarian cancer found that women who habitually consumed animal fats and saturated fats increased the risk of ovarian cancer by 70% and 24%, respectively.

• Conclusion

The meta-analytical results revealed that consumption of animal fats increased the risk of the incidences of breast cancer, endometrial cancer, and ovarian cancer (see Table 31.3). Women who consumed animal fats were found to increase the risk of breast cancer, endometrial cancer, and ovarian cancer by 15%, 17%, and 70%, respectively.

In brief, high consumption of animal fats is associated with an increased risk of gynecological cancers, particularly ovarian cancer. Women should avoid eating foods that are high in animal fats, such as beef, lamb, fried chicken, sausages, bacon, and ham.

Table 31.3. Meta-analytical Confirmation of Animal Fat Consumption Associated with an Increased Risk of Gynecological Cancers

Gynecological Cancers	Increased Risk, Animal Fats
Breast cancer	Animal fats increased the risk of breast cancer by 15%.
Endometrial cancer	Daily consumption of 5 g and 10 g of animal fats increased the risk of endometrial cancer by 5% and 17%, respectively in women on a daily 1,000 calorie diet.
Ovarian cancer	High consumption of animal fats and saturated fats increased the risk of ovarian cancer by 70% and 24%, respectively. Daily consumption of 30 g of animal fats increased the risk of ovarian cancer by 17%.

• Recommendation

Prevention — Every woman, particularly for those who are at risk of gynecological cancers and gynecological cancer patients, should avoid consuming foods that are high in animal fats or saturated fats.

32

Processed Meat

Processed meat refers to any meat preserved by smoking, curing, salting, or adding preservatives, such as nitrites and nitrates. Sausages, hot dogs, bacon, ham, salami, and beef jerky are common processed meat. The history of processed meat dates back 3,000 years ago; historical records have revealed that the ancient Chinese and Greeks preserved meats with salt, and in the Roman times, people noted that adding nitrates changed their meat to a reddish color. Despite significant strides and advances in the modern food industry, the most commonly used food preservatives are still nitrites and nitrates.

Why can processed meat be harmful to health?

- High sodium — Processed meat has high contents of sodium, which raise blood sodium concentrations, leading to hypertension and increasing the risk of stroke.
- Animal fats — Processed meats such as bacon, hot dogs, and sausages contain a high amount of animal fats. Once absorbed by the intestines, these excessive animal fats are likely stored in adipose tissues in various regions of the body, which can contribute to becoming overweight and the risk of obesity.
- Carcinogens — During roasting, frying or preserving stage, processed meat can generate carcinogenic compounds such as nitrosamine compounds, heterocyclic amines, and polycyclic aromatic hydrocarbons. These carcinogenic compounds can damage the DNA and increase the risk of cancers. The International

Agency for Research on Cancer, the cancer research agency of World Health Organization, has recommended that processed meat be considered as Group 1 human carcinogens.

- Nitrites — Nitrites and nitrates are preservatives found in processed meat. These preservatives can react with meat proteins to give rise to carcinogenic nitrosamine compounds and elevate the risk of cancers. Nitrosamine compounds are also harmful to the pancreas, diminishing insulin secretion, and elevating the risk of type 2 diabetes.

What Types of Chronic Disease can be Caused by Consuming Processed Meat?

• Meta-analysis

Breast cancer — Women who frequently consume processed meat have an increased risk of breast cancer.

Twelve prospective studies on the association between processed meat consumption and breast cancer found that each additional serving of processed meat per day increased the risk of breast cancer by 9%.

Colorectal adenomas — People who consume processed meat (two ounces daily) significantly elevate the risk of colorectal adenomas.

A meta-analysis of 26 clinical reports investigated the relationship between processed meat and colorectal adenomas showed that a daily consumption of 50 g of processed meat increased the risk of colorectal adenomas by 29%.

Esophageal cancer — High consumption of processed meat can lead to esophageal cancer.

Twenty-one clinical trials on the association between processed meat consumption and esophageal cancer including 6,499 esophageal cancer cases revealed that consumption of processed meat increased the risk of esophageal cancer by 55%.

Heart disease — High consumption of processed meat hastens the incidence of coronary heart disease and heart failure.

Nine prospective studies evaluated the relationship between processed meat consumption and heart disease including 23,889 coronary heart disease cases found that a daily consumption of 50 g of processed meat increased the risk of coronary heart disease by 42%. People who consume two ounces of processed meat daily greatly increase the risk of coronary heart disease. Another meta-analysis of 123 prospective studies on the association between processed meat and heart disease revealed that consumption of processed meat increased the risk of coronary heart disease by 27% and the risk of heart failure by 12%.

Lung cancer — Consuming processed meat (two ounces daily) significantly heightens the risk of lung cancer.

A meta-analysis of 34 clinical studies on the relationship between processed meat and lung cancer found that consumption of processed meat increased the risk of lung cancer by 23%. The dose-response analysis showed that each additional intake of 50 g of processed meat per day increased the risk of lung cancer by 20%.

Oral cancer — Habitual consumption of processed meat can cause oral cancer.

Thirteen research articles investigated the relationship between processed meat consumption and oral cancer reported that high processed meat consumption increased the risk of oral cancer by 91%.

Pancreatic cancer — People who consume processed meat (two ounces daily) have discernibly increased risks of pancreatic cancer.

Eleven prospective studies on the association between processed meat intake and pancreatic cancer showed that each additional intake of 50 g of processed meat per day increased the risk of pancreatic cancer by 19%.

Premature mortality — Consumption of processed meat (two ounces daily) noticeably augments the risk of premature mortality.

A meta-analysis of 17 prospective studies on the relationship between processed meat consumption and premature mortality including 150,328 all-cause mortality cases found that each additional serving of processed meat per day increased the risk of all-cause mortality, cardiovascular disease mortality, and cancer mortality by 15%, 15%, and 8%, respectively. In other words, high consumption of processed meat greatly elevated the risk of premature mortalities from cardiovascular disease and cancer. Another meta-analysis of 12 prospective studies on the relationship between processed meat consumption and premature mortality revealed that each additional intake of 50 g of processed meat per day increased the risk of all-cause mortality by 23%.

Stomach cancer — Habitual consumption of ham and sausages greatly increases the risk of stomach cancer.

A meta-analysis of 57 prospective studies examined the association between process meat consumption and stomach cancer found that high consumption of processed meat increased the risk of stomach cancer by 76%. Analysis confirms that high consumption of processed meat could lead to stomach cancer. Another meta-analysis of 30 clinical studies on the relationship between processed meat consumption and stomach cancer showed that ham and sausage consumption increased the risk of stomach cancer by 44% and 33%, respectively.

Stroke — Consumption of processed meat (two ounces daily) worsens the risk of stroke.

A meta-analysis of seven prospective studies evaluated the association between processed meat and stroke revealed that regular consumption of processed meat increased the risk of total stroke by 17%, which confirms that people who regularly consumed processed meat significantly heightened the risk of stroke. Another meta-analysis of five prospective studies on the relationship between processed meat and stroke found that processed meat increased the risk of total stroke by 14% and the risk of ischemic stroke by 19%. In addition, each additional intake of 50 g of processed meat increased the risk of stroke by 11%.

Type 2 diabetes — Daily consumption of processed meat (two ounces) significantly heightens the risk of type 2 diabetes.

Fourteen prospective studies evaluated the association between processed meat and type 2 diabetes reported that a daily consumption of 50 g of processed meat increased the fasting glucose level by 0.38 mg/dL. In brief, people who consume two ounces of processed meat per day can raise fasting blood glucose levels and elevate the risk of type 2 diabetes. Another meta-analysis of three prospective studies on the relationship between processed meat consumption and type 2 diabetes found that each additional serving of processed meat daily increased the risk of type 2 diabetes by 32%. The dose-response analysis revealed that each additional intake of 50 g of processed meat daily increased the risk of type 2 diabetes by 51%. In short, consuming processed meat could greatly increase the incidence of type 2 diabetes. Further supporting evidence about harmful effects of processed meat, a meta-analysis of nine prospective studies including 10,797 type 2 diabetes cases found that each additional intake of 50 g of processed meat daily increased the risk of type 2 diabetes by 19%.

• Conclusion

The meta-analytic studies showed that consumption of processed meat increased the risk of chronic diseases, including stroke, coronary heart disease, type 2 diabetes, breast cancer, oral cancer, esophageal cancer, stomach cancer, lung cancer, pancreatic cancer, colorectal cancer as well as premature mortality (see Table 32.1). Specifically, the data revealed that consuming processed meat increased the risk of all strokes, ischemic stroke, and coronary heart disease by 14%, 19%, and 27%, respectively. It is worth mentioning that processed meat increased the risk of type 2 diabetes by 32%. In addition, consuming processed meat increased the risk of oral

Table 32.1. Meta-analytical Confirmation of Processed Meat Consumption Associated with an Increased Risk of Chronic Diseases and Premature Mortality

Chronic Diseases	Increased Risk, Processed Meat
Breast cancer	Women who regularly consumed processed meat increased the risk of breast cancer by 9%.
Colorectal adenomas	Daily consumption of 50 g of processed meat increased the risk of colorectal adenomas by 29%.
Esophageal cancer	Processed meat increased the risk of esophageal cancer by 55%.
Heart disease	Processed meat increased the risk of coronary heart disease by 27% and heart failure by 12%. Daily intake of 50 g of processed meat increased coronary heart disease by 42%.
Lung cancer	Processed meat increased the risk of lung cancer by 23%. Each additional intake of 50 g of processed meat per day increased the risk of lung cancer by 20%.
Oral cancer	Processed meat increased the risk of oral cancer by 91%.
Pancreatic cancer	Each additional intake of 50 g of processed meat per day increased the risk of pancreatic cancer by 19%.
Premature mortality	Each additional serving of processed meat per day increased the risk of all-cause mortality, cardiovascular disease mortality, and cancer mortality by 15%, 15%, and 8%, respectively. Each additional intake of 50 g of processed meat per day increased the risk of all-cause mortality by 23%.
Stomach cancer	Processed meat increased the risk of stomach cancer by 76%. Consumption of ham and sausages increased the risk of stomach cancer by 44% and 33%, respectively.
Stroke	Processed meat increased the risk of total stroke and ischemic stroke by 14–17% and 19%, respectively. Additional intake of 50 g of processed meat per day increased the risk of stroke by 11%.
Type 2 diabetes	Additional intake of 50 g of processed meat per day increased fasting glucose level by 0.38 mg/dL. Each additional intake of 50 g of processed meat per day increased the risk of type 2 diabetes by 19%.

cancer, esophageal cancer, and colorectal cancer by 91%, 55%, and 29%, respectively. When analyzed one at a time, consumption of bacon, ham, and sausages has been found to increase the risk of stomach cancer by 37%, 44%, and 33%, respectively. Finally, processed meat increased the risk of all-cause mortality, cardiovascular disease mortality, and cancer mortality by 15%, 15%, and 8%, respectively.

In conclusion, consumption of processed meat is associated with an increased risk of type 2 diabetes and stroke, and cardiovascular disease as well as the risk of breast cancer, lung cancer, and gastrointestinal cancers, such as oral cancer, esophageal cancer, stomach cancer, pancreatic cancer, and colorectal cancer. In addition, processed meat consumption also has an increased risk of premature mortality.

• Recommendation

Prevention — Everyone, especially for those who are at risk of chronic disease and chronic disease patients, should avoid consuming any processed meat.

What Types of Chronic Disease can be Caused by Consuming both Red Meat and Processed Meat?

Red meat and processed meat, which consist of 58% and 22% of total daily meat consumption in the United States, are a substantial part of American diet. We have previously talked about consuming red meat or processed meat alone associated with an increased risk of chronic diseases. Most people who like steak, often also like bacon and sausages. So, what is the relationship between combined consumption of red meat and processed meat and the risk of chronic diseases?

• Meta-analysis

Breast cancer — Women who consume red meat and processed meat daily have an increased risk of breast cancer.

Eight prospective studies on the association between red meat and processed meat consumption and breast cancer found that each additional serving of red meat and processed meat per day increased the risk of breast cancer by 7%.

Colorectal adenomas — High consumption of red meat and processed meat begets the risk of colorectal adenomas.

Sixteen clinical reports examined the association between red meat and processed meat consumption and colorectal adenomas showed that consumption of red and processed meat increased the risk of colorectal adenomas by 29%.

Colorectal cancer — High consumption of red meat and processed meat augments the risk of colorectal cancer.

Another meta-analysis of 16 clinical studies on the relationship between red meat and processed meat consumption and colorectal cancer revealed that consumption of red meat and processed meat increased the risk of colorectal cancer by 29%.

Oral cancer — People who regularly consume red meat and processed meat exacerbate the incidence of oral cancer.

Thirteen research articles evaluated the association between red meat and processed meat consumption and oral cancer found that consumption of red meat and processed meat increased the risk of oral cancer by 14%.

Premature mortality — Regular consumption of red meat and processed meat fosters the risk of premature mortality.

Nine prospective studies on the relationship between red meat and processed meat consumption and premature mortality revealed that consumption of red meat and processed meat was found to increase the risk of all-cause mortality by 29%.

Stroke — People who consume red meat and processed meat daily have an elevated risk of stroke.

A meta-analysis of seven prospective studies on the association between red meat and processed meat consumption and stroke showed that consumption of red meat and processed meat increased the risk of total stroke, cerebral infarction, and ischemic stroke by 14%, 13%, and 22%, respectively. Analysis evinces that high consumption of red meat and processed meat could augment the incidence of stroke. Another meta-analysis of six prospective studies investigated the relationship between red meat and processed meat consumption and stroke found that each additional serving of red meat and processed meat increased the risk of stroke by 11%.

• Conclusion

The meta-analysis data confirms that combined consumption of red meat and processed meat increased the risk of stroke, breast cancer, colorectal cancer, and premature mortality (see Table 32.2). Consumption of red meat and processed meat has been found to increase the risk of all strokes and ischemic stroke by 14% and 22%, respectively. For women, red meat and processed meat increased the risk of breast cancer by 7%. Not surprisingly, consuming red meat and processed meat has been found to increase the risk of

Table 32.2. **Meta-analytical Confirmation of Combined Consumption of Red Meat and Processed Meat Associated with an Increased Risk of Chronic Diseases and of Premature Mortality**

Chronic Diseases	Increased Risk, Red Meat and Processed Meat
Breast cancer	Each additional serving of red meat and processed meat per day increased by the risk of breast cancer by 7%.
Colorectal adenomas	Red meat and processed meat increased the risk of colorectal adenomas by 29%.
Colorectal cancer	Red meat and processed meat increased the risk of colorectal cancer by 29%.
Oral cancer	Red meat and processed meat increased the risk of oral cancer by 14%.
Premature mortality	Red meat and processed meat increased the risk of all-cause mortality by 29%.

colorectal cancer by 29%. Moreover, high consumption of red meat and processed meat increased the risk of all-cause mortality by 29%.

In summary, combined consumption of red meat and processed meat is associated with higher incident rates of stroke and cancers, including breast cancer and colorectal cancer, as well as the risk of premature mortality.

• Recommendation

Prevention — People at risk of chronic diseases should not consume more than 4 ounces of red meat per week and should not consume any processed meat. Chronic disease patients should avoid consuming any red meat or processed meat.

33

Sugar-sweetened Beverages

Before the 15th century, sugar consumption per capita was zero throughout the world. Southeast Asia was the only place in the world where people cultivated sugar canes. In the mid-16th century, Portuguese sailors invaded Southeast Asia and recognized the economic potential of sugar cane. They brought sugar canes from Southeast Asia to the Caribbean islands where they used African slave labor to operate large-scale sugar cane plantations. By the end of the 17th century, sugar had become a favorable condiment of European noble families. During the time of the Revolutionary War in the United States, sugar consumption per capita was about 18 pounds per capita, and it increased to about 60 pounds per capita during the 19th century. To date, an average American consumes about 100 pounds of sugar per year, which is equivalent to 126 g or 32 teaspoons of sugar per day. The American Heart Association recommends a daily intake of 39 g of sugar per day for men and 24 g per day for women. Americans consume three times more sugar than the amount deemed healthy by the American Heart Association.

What types of processed food contain the highest sugar contents?

In the US grocery stores, about 74% of all processed food items are laced with sugar. Food manufacturers have used more than 66 different names for sugar, some of which are scientific names that are beyond comprehension by laymen. Therefore, people often purchase processed foods without knowing their actual sugar contents.

In addition, among all nutritional facts listed on the food label, sugar is the only nutrient that displays only the amount; it does not show the % Daily Value. Hence, when consuming processed foods, you have no way of knowing your total daily sugar intake compared to the amount recommended by the United States FDA or the American Heart Association. Consequently, most people probably consume much more sugar than they ever realize.

Table 33.1 depicts the sugar contents of some common food items, for example, a glass of chocolate milk contains 52 g of sugar, a slice of fruit cake contains 43 g of sugar, and a can of soda contains 39 g of sugar. Since Americans regularly consume these processed foods, it is therefore of no surprise that sugar consumption is three times higher than the recommended daily intake.

Table 33.1.   Sugar Contents in Some Common Food Items

Food Items (100 g)	Sucrose Contents G	Total Sugar Contents (including Sucrose and Non-sucrose Sugar) g
Chocolate milk	46.8	52.1
Chocolate sauce	30.5	51.8
Wheat popcorn, sugar-laced	38.0	45.1
Root beer	20.7	44.0
Fruit cake	20.5	43.1
Corn-flakes, sugar-laced	37.6	39.6
Soda	7.8	39.2
Popcorn, sugar-laced	37.7	39.0
Fruit pie	21.5	30.9
Chocolate chips	22.2	25.0
Strawberry smoothie	1.5	18.6
Vanilla milkshake	1.0	17.8
Chocolate milkshake	0.9	17.6
Strawberry yogurt	0.7	15.3

*Data adapted from the 1987 USDA sources.

Why is sugar harmful to health?

Sugar-sweetened beverages account for 9.2% of the total daily calorie intake per capita in the United States. Sugar that is added to sugar-sweetened beverages is almost 100% absorbed by the intestines, which leads to high blood glucose levels. In response to that, the pancreas secrets insulin, a hormone that acts like a key to allow sugar to enter the cells in the body, and thus lowers blood sugar level. Habitual consumption of sugar-sweetened beverages causes the pancreas to incessantly secret a large amount of insulin, which blunts cellular responses to insulin and gives rise to insulin resistance. Insulin resistance is the causative factor for a host of chronic diseases including obesity, hypertension, hypercholesterolemia, chronic pancreatic disease, cognitive impairment, and even cancers. Alzheimer's disease is a form of brain insulin resistance, a condition in which the neurons are unable to absorb and utilize glucose, which results in neuronal death. That is why Alzheimer's disease is also called "type 3 diabetes".

In addition, habitual consumption of sugar-sweetened beverages can raise blood level of C-reactive protein, which can increase the risk of atherosclerosis and coronary heart disease. Moreover, sugar-sweetened beverages can elevate the blood levels of uric acid, cause endothelial dysfunction, and reduce the production of nitric oxide. Insufficient production of nitric oxide can lead to hypertension and atherosclerosis and augment the incidence of coronary heart disease.

What Types of Chronic Disease can be Caused by Drinking Sugar-Sweetened Beverages?

• Meta-analysis

Chronic kidney disease — High consumption of sugar-sweetened beverages can lead to chronic kidney disease.

Five prospective studies on the relationship between consumption of sugar-sweetened beverages and chronic kidney disease found that consumption of sugar-sweetened beverages increased the risk of chronic kidney disease by 58%.

Heart disease — High consumption of sugar-sweetened beverages aggravates the risk of heart disease (coronary heart disease and myocardial infarction).

A meta-analysis of four prospective studies investigated the association between sugar-sweetened beverage consumption and heart disease included a total of 173,753 participants, of which 7,396 were coronary heart disease cases. The results showed that each additional sugar-sweetened beverage consumed daily increased the risk of coronary heart disease by 16%. In other words, habitual consumption of sugar-sweetened beverages heightened the risk of coronary heart disease. Additional supporting evidence about the harmful effects of sugar-sweetened beverages is presented in the meta-analysis of seven prospective studies in 308,420 people, which showed that consumption of sugar-sweetened beverages increased the risk of myocardial infarction by 19%.

Hypercholesterolemia — High consumption of fructose exacerbates blood cholesterol levels in patients with hypercholesterolemia.

Twenty-four controlled-feeding clinical studies on the relationship between fructose consumption and hypercholesterolemia revealed that daily consumption of 100 g of fructose increased the LDL cholesterol level by 11.6 mg/dL and triglycerides by 13.0 mg/dL.

Hypertension — Daily consumption of sugar-sweetened beverages elevates blood pressure in pre-hypertensive individuals and patients with hypertension.

Nine prospective studies examined the association between sugar-sweetened beverages and hypertension included 240,508 participants, of which 79,251 were hypertensive patients. The results showed that consumption of sugar-sweetened beverages increased a person's risk of developing hypertension by 12%. The dose-response data showed that each additional serving of sugar-sweetened beverages per day increased the risk of hypertension by 8%.

Obesity — High consumption of sugar-sweetened beverages increases the risk of obesity.

A meta-analysis of 15 prospective studies on the relationship between sugar-sweetened beverages and obesity in 11,703 people found that frequent consumption of sugar-sweetened beverages increased 0.85 kg in body weight. The dose-response analysis showed that each additional intake of 1 can of sugar-sweetened beverages daily increased body weight by 0.22 kg. In brief, daily consumption of sugar-sweetened beverages augmented the risk of obesity. Another meta-analysis of three prospective studies evaluated the association between sugar-sweetened beverages and obesity revealed that habitual consumption of sugar-sweetened beverages increased the risk of obesity by 18%.

Type 2 diabetes — People who consume sugar-sweetened beverages (1 can daily) have greater risks of type 2 diabetes.

Seventeen prospective studies on the relationship between consumption of sugar-sweetened beverages and type 2 diabetes including 38,253 type 2 diabetes cases showed that each additional serving of sugar-sweetened beverages daily increased the risk of type 2 diabetes by 13%. The studies forecasted that additional 2 million Americans and 80,000 British people will suffer from type 2 diabetes in the next 10 years, because of the increased consumption of sugar-sweetened beverages in these two countries. Another meta-analysis of 11 prospective studies on the association of sugar-sweetened beverages and type 2 diabetes included a total of 310,819 participants, of which 12,375 were type 2 diabetes cases. The results revealed that a daily consumption of 1–2 cans of sugar-sweetened beverages increased the risk of type 2 diabetes by 26%. In other words, daily consumption of sugar-sweetened beverages greatly raises the risk of type 2 diabetes. Further supporting evidence about the harmful effects of sugar-sweetened beverages is documented in a meta-analysis of nine prospective studies, which showed that a daily consumption of 330 ml of sugar-sweetened beverages increased the risk of type 2 diabetes by 20%.

• Conclusion

The meta-analytical data has demonstrated that consuming sugar-sweetened beverages increased the risk of obesity, hypertension, hypercholesterolemia, type 2 diabetes, heart disease, and chronic kidney disease (see Table 33.2). Specifically, consuming sugar-sweetened beverages increased the risk of obesity, hypertension, and type 2 diabetes by 18%, 12%, and 13%, respectively.

Table 33.2. Meta-analytical Confirmation of Consumption of Sugar-sweetened Beverages Associated with Higher Risks of Chronic Diseases

Chronic Diseases	Increased Risk, Sugar-sweetened Beverages
Chronic kidney disease	Sugar-sweetened beverages increased the risk of chronic kidney disease by 58%.
Heart disease	Sugar-sweetened beverages increased the risk of coronary heart disease and myocardial infarction by 16% and 19%, respectively.
Hypercholesterolemia	Daily intake of 100 g of fructose increased LDL cholesterol by 11.6 mg/dL and triglycerides by 13.0 mg/dL.
Hypertension	Sugar-sweetened increased the risk of hypertension by 12%.
Obesity	Sugar-sweetened beverages increased weight gain by 1.9 lbs. Each additional intake of one can of sugar-sweetened beverage per day increased weight gain by 0.5 lb.
Type 2 diabetes	Sugar-sweetened beverages increased the risk of type 2 diabetes by 13%. Each additional intake of 1–2 cans of sugar-sweetened beverages per day increased the risk of type 2 diabetes by 26%. Each additional intake of 300 ml of sugar-sweetened beverages per day increased the risk of type 2 diabetes by 20%.

In hypercholesterolemic patients, consuming sugar-sweetened beverages increased LDL cholesterol by 11.6 mg/dL and triglycerides by 13.0 mg/dL. People who habitually drank sugar-sweetened beverages increased the risk of coronary heart disease, myocardial infarction, and chronic kidney disease by 16%, 19%, and 58%, respectively.

In summary, consuming sugar-sweetened beverages is associated with elevated risks of obesity, type 2 diabetes and hypertension, and exacerbates blood lipid profiles in hypercholesterolemic patients. In addition, consuming sugar-sweetened beverages is associated with higher risks of cardiovascular disease and chronic kidney disease.

• Recommendation

Prevention — Everyone, particularly for those who are at risk of chronic diseases and chronic disease patients should avoid consuming any sugar-sweetened beverage.

34

Artificially-sweetened Beverages

Saccharin, aspartame, sucralose, acesulfame, and neotame are five commonly used artificial sweeteners found in beverages and processed foods. These artificial sweeteners are 200–400 times sweeter than sucrose. Adding only a small quantity of the artificial sweetener is enough to achieve the desired sweet taste in beverages; yet it provides no added nutritional values or benefits. Besides beverages, artificially sweeteners are also found in a multitude of products including chewing gums, toothpaste, processed foods, and medicine.

What Types of Chronic Disease is Caused by Artificially Sweetened Beverages?

• Meta-analysis

Hypertension — Habitual consumption of artificially-sweetened beverages augments the risk of hypertension.

Twelve prospective studies on the association between artificially-sweetened beverage consumption and hypertension found that consumption of artificially sweetened beverages increased the risk of hypertension by 15%.

Obesity — High consumption of artificially sweetened beverages can lead to obesity.

A meta-analysis of three prospective studies examined the relationship between artificially-sweetened beverage consumption and obesity showed that habitual consumption of artificially sweetened beverages increased the risk of obesity by 59%.

Stroke — People who regularly consume artificially-sweetened beverages have a noticeably elevated risk of stroke.

Seven prospective studies on the association between artificially-sweetened beverage consumption and stroke in 308,420 people revealed that high consumption of artificially sweetened beverages increased the risk of stroke by 14%.

Type 2 diabetes — Daily consumption of artificially-sweetened beverages hastens the risk of type 2 diabetes.

A meta-analysis of 17 prospective studies evaluated the relationship between artificially-sweetened beverages and type 2 diabetes found that each additional serving of artificially-sweetened beverages daily increased the risk of type 2 diabetes by 8%.

• Conclusion

The meta-analytical results have revealed that consumption of artificially-sweetened beverages increased the risk of obesity, hypertension, type 2 diabetes, stroke, and cardiovascular disease.

Table 34.1. Meta-analytical Confirmation of Consumption of Artificially-sweetened Beverages Associated with an Increased Risk of Chronic Diseases

Chronic Diseases	Increased Risk, Artificially-sweetened Beverages
Hypertension	Artificially-sweetened beverages increased the risk of hypertension by 15%.
Obesity	Artificially-sweetened beverages increased the risk of obesity by 59%.
Stroke	Artificially-sweetened beverages increased the risk of stroke by 14%.
Type 2 diabetes	Each additional serving of artificially-sweetened beverages per day increased the risk of type 2 diabetes by 8%.

As shown in Table 34.1, consumption of artificially-sweetened beverages has been found to increase the risk of obesity, hypertension, type 2 diabetes, and stroke by 59%, 15%, 8%, and 14%, respectively.

In summary, habitually drinking artificially-sweetened beverages are just as harmful to health as habitually drinking sugar-sweetened beverages.

• **Recommendation**

Prevention — Everyone, especially for those who are at risk of chronic diseases and chronic disease patients should avoid consuming any artificially-sweetened beverages.

35

High Glycemic-load Foods

High glycemic-load foods include white rice, white bread, potatoes, spaghetti, flour tortillas, and bagels. Among these high glycemic-load foods, white rice is a staple food of Asians, while white bread, potatoes, spaghetti, macaroni, and pizza are staple foods of Westerners and favorable foods worldwide.

What is the glycemic index?

Glycemic index (GI) is a numeric ranking that measures how foods affect the blood glucose level within 2 to 3 hours after eating. Pure glucose has a GI value of 100. The glycemic indexes of food items range from 0 to 100 with 0–55 = low-GI, 56–69 = medium-GI, and 70–100 = high-GI. A high-GI food item implies that ingestion of this food can rapidly increase blood glucose levels like that of glucose. On the other hand, a low-GI food implies that ingestion of this food will not affect blood glucose levels. Glycemic indexes of most food items lie between 20 and 80. Habitual intake of high GI foods can lead to chronic diseases such as type 2 diabetes, while habitual intake of low GI foods may prevent chronic diseases.

Although the concept of the glycemic index is very simple, it does have its limitations. Glycemic index emphasizes the food's effect on the blood glucose level, but it does not account for the quantity of the food consumed. For instance, eating a small amount of a high-GI food will only have a minor effect on the blood glucose level, but eating a large amount of a moderate-GI food will cause an instant increase in the blood glucose level. Therefore, it is important to consider not only the type of food but also the quantity of food when measuring the impact of food on blood glucose levels. The concept of glycemic load was created to resolve the shortcomings of the glycemic index.

What is glycemic load?

Foods generally contain proteins, lipids, and carbohydrates, of which only carbohydrates can affect blood glucose level. Glycemic load (GL) accounts for the glycemic index of a given food item plus its carbohydrate content. To calculate glycemic load, multiply the glycemic index of a food item by its carbohydrate content and then divide by 100. Foods with a glycemic load of 10 or lower are called low glycemic load foods (low-GL foods) and foods with a glycemic load of 11 and 19 are called moderate glycemic load foods (moderate-GL foods). Food items with a glycemic load value higher than 20 are considered high glycemic load foods (high-GL foods), which can readily raise blood glucose levels. As previously mentioned, white rice, white bread, potatoes, spaghetti, flour tortillas, and bagels are high-GL foods. Frequent consumption of these foods may lead to high blood glucose, weight gain, insulin resistance, and type 2 diabetes.

It is important to note that the glycemic index of food item is a fixed number, but the glycemic load of a food item is not a fixed number. In other words, the glycemic index serves for comparison purposes, while the glycemic load is more useful in daily dietary consideration. For example, the glycemic index of white rice is 72, and a bowl of white rice weights about 150 g and contains 40.3 g of carbohydrate. Based on this information, we can easily calculate that the glycemic load of one bowl of white rice is 29 (72 times 40.3, divides by 100) and the glycemic load of one-half bowl of white rice is 14.5, while the glycemic load of two bowls of white rice is 58. As we have discussed previously, foods with glycemic load of 20 or higher are high-GL foods. Consuming one-half bowl of white rice a day may only have a moderate effect on blood glucose level but consuming more than one bowl of white rice each day can lead to high blood glucose and the risk of type 2 diabetes.

Glycemic load of some common food items

Table 35.1 illustrates the glycemic load values of some common food items. High-GL food items include potatoes, white rice, raisins, bagels, macaroni, sweet potatoes, spaghetti, and corn, and low-GL food items include vegetables, legumes, fruits, and nuts. The glycemic load values of potatoes and white rice are 33 and 29, respectively. High consumption of potatoes, white rice, or other high-GL food items can increase blood glucose levels, insulin resistance, and the risk of type 2 diabetes. Diabetic patients and other chronic disease patients should avoid eating any high-GL food items. Whole grains, vegetables, fruits, nuts, legumes, and milk are low-GL foods; consumption of these foods will reduce the risk of chronic diseases, including type 2 diabetes.

Why is high glycemic-load food harmful to health?

High glycemic-load foods include white bread and white rice. White rice is the staple food of more than one half of whole world population. The glycemic index of white rice is 72, compared to 50 for brown rice, 55 for oats, and 45 for wheat. Consumption of white rice can elevate the risk of type 2 diabetes because of its high glycemic index. In addition, white rice, which contains only the endosperm without the bran and germ, lacks many nutrients, vitamins, and essential elements. People who habitually consume white rice are likely to have vitamin and nutrient insufficiencies, resulting in weak immune system and poor metabolic health.

Habitual consumption of high glycemic-load foods can also increase insulin-like growth factor and the risk of insulin resistance. Insulin-like growth factor can stimulate the ovary to produce estrogen hormones, trigger the growth and proliferation of cancerous cells in the uterus, and increase the risk of endometrial cancer. Insulin resistance is a causative factor for many chronic diseases, including type 2 diabetes and cancers.

Table 35.1. Glycemic Index (GI) and Glycemic Load (GL) Values of Some Common Food Items

Food Items	Glycemic Index (GI)	Intake, g	Carbohydrate Content, g	Glycemic Load (GL)
High-GL food items				
Potato	111	150	29.7	33
White rice	72	150	40.3	29
Raisins	64	60	43.8	28
Bagel	72	70	34.7	25
Macaroni	50	180	48.0	24
Sweet potato	70	150	31.4	22
Spaghetti	46	180	47.8	22
Corn-flakes	81	30	24.7	20
Moderate-GL food items				
Coca Cola	63	250 ml	25.4	16
Brown rice	50	150	32.0	16
Whole wheat	45	50	33.3	15
Corn	48	60	17.9	14
Quinoa	53	150	24.5	13
Oatmeal	55	250	23.6	13
Corn tortilla	52	50	23.1	12
Grape juice	41	250 ml	29.3	12
Orange juice	50	250 ml	24	12
White bread	75	30	14.7	11
Banana	48	120	22.9	11
Red grapes	59	120	18.6	11
Low-GL food items				
Pita	68	30	14.7	10
Whole wheat bread	69	30	13.0	9
Ice cream	62	50	12.9	8
Wheat cake	30	50	26.7	8
Hamburger buns	61	30	11.5	7

Table 35.1. (*Continued*)

Food Items	Glycemic Index (GI)	Intake, g	Carbohydrate Content, g	Glycemic Load (GL)
Black bean	30	150	23.3	7
Lentils	28	150	17.9	5
Apple	36	120	13.9	5
Orange	45	120	11.1	5
Whole milk	31	250 ml	12.9	4
Watermelon	72	120	5.6	4
Green bean	54	80	7.4	4
Tomato juice	38	250 ml	10.5	4
Pistachio nut	22	50	13.6	3
Carrots	39	80	5.1	2
Soybean	15	150	6.7	1
Peanut	13	50	7.7	1

Fiona S *et al.*, *Diabetes Care*, 2008, **31**(12); 2281–2283.

What Types of Chronic Disease can be Caused by Consuming High Glycemic-Load Foods?

• Meta-analysis

Colorectal cancer — Habitual consumption of high glycemic-load foods greatly exacerbates the risk of colorectal cancer.

Thirty-nine research articles studied the association between consumption of high glycemic-load foods and colorectal cancer found that consumption of high glycemic-load foods increased the risk of colorectal cancer by **26%**.

Endometrial cancer — Women who consume high glycemic-load foods (two ounces daily) significantly increases the risk of endometrial cancer.

Five epidemiological studies on high glycemic-load foods and endometrial cancer showed that consumption of high glycemic-load foods increased the risk of endometrial cancer by **20%** in pre- and postmenopausal women. Furthermore, obese women who consumed high glycemic-load foods increased the risk of endometrial cancer by 54%. Put it simply, women who habitually consume high glycemic-load foods can lead to the incidence of endometrial cancer. Another meta-analysis of eight research papers evaluated the relationship between consumption of high glycemic-load foods and endometrial cancer revealed that each additional intake of 50 units of glycemic load foods increased the risk of endometrial cancer by 21%. (Note: One unit of glycemic-load food gives rise to the glycemic effect of 1 g of glucose.)

Type 2 diabetes — Daily consumption of white rice can greatly increase the risk of type 2 diabetes, particularly in Asians.

Seven prospective studies on white rice consumption and type 2 diabetes in 352,384 participants including 13,284 type 2 diabetes cases showed that a daily consumption of white rice increased the risk of type 2 diabetes by 55% in Asian people and the risk of type 2 diabetes by 12% in Western people. Each additional serving of white rice per day increased the risk of type 2 diabetes by 11%.

• Conclusion

The meta-analytic results confirm that consuming high-GL foods significantly increased the risk of type 2 diabetes, endometrial cancer, and colorectal cancer (see Table 35.2). Specifically, high

Table 35.2. Meta-analytical Confirmation of Consumption of High Glycemic-load Foods Associated with an Increased Risk of Chronic Diseases

Chronic Diseases	Increased Risk, High-GL Foods
Colorectal cancer	White rice increased the risk of colorectal cancer by 26%.
Endometrial cancer	High-GL foods increased the risk of endometrial cancer in normal weight women and obese women by 20% and 54%, respectively.
Type 2 diabetes	White rice consumption increased the risk of type 2 diabetes in Asians and Westerners by 55% and 12%, respectively.

consumption of white rice has been found to increase the risk of type 2 diabetes by 55%. In addition, women who consumed high-GL foods increased the risk of endometrial cancer by 20%, and obese women who consumed high-GL foods increased the risk of endometrial cancer by 54%. Furthermore, consumption of high-GL foods raised the risk of colorectal cancer by 26%.

In conclusion, the habitual intake of high-GL foods is associated with higher incident rates of type 2 diabetes, colorectal cancer, and endometrial cancer.

• Recommendation

Prevention — People who are at risk of chronic diseases and chronic disease patients should avoid consuming any high glycemic-load foods such as white rice, white bread, spaghetti, and the like.

36

High-Salt Foods

The chemical formula of table salt is sodium chloride. In water, sodium chloride instantly dissociates to a sodium ion and a chloride ion, both of which are important chemical elements for the human body. Sodium ion is involved in a multitude of physiological functions, including regulating blood pressure, membrane potential, and membrane permeability. Nevertheless, a high-salt diet can be harmful to health because it can lead to chronic diseases:

- Hypertension — High blood sodium level causes the outflow of intracellular water into the blood stream, which expands blood volume, exerts extra pressure against vessel wall, and leads to hypertension.
- Immune function — High-salt intake diminishes immune function and makes the body more susceptible to infections. Individuals with familial autoimmune diseases who consume salty foods are known to exacerbate the condition of the disease.
- Cardiovascular system — High-salt intake can thicken the chamber wall of the left ventricle in the heart and hardens the wall of blood vessels, which increases the risk of heart disease and stroke.
- Liver — A high-salt diet damages liver cells, causes liver fibrosis, and diminishes hepatic functions. Harmful effects of high salt on the liver are likely mediated by free radicals. Foods rich in

Vitamin C can neutralize free radicals and attenuate salt-related oxidative damage to the liver.

What types of foods have high salt contents?

During a meal, we often pay more attention to the taste of the food than the content of the food. Because of that, most people tend to eat more salt than they realize, and over time develop an unhealthy dietary habit of assuming that salted food is delicious and unsalted food is bland. Table 36.1 depicts the salt content of 15 common processed food items. Taken the data from Table 36.1, if you eat two pieces of bacon for breakfast (4.9 g salt), one hamburger for lunch (3.3 g salt), and some cheese and ham for dinner (7.0 g salt), your salt intake will already be 15 g for the day. The American

Table 36.1. A List of Processed Foods with High-salt Content

Food Items	Amount, g	Sodium Content, g	Salt Content, g
Bacon	40	1.87	4.9
Salami	90	1.85	4.8
Olives, salted	20	1.80	4.7
Cheese	25	1.41	3.7
Beef hamburger	170	1.25	3.3
Ham	90	1.25	3.3
Corn-flakes	30	1.17	3.1
Sausage, beef	120	1.09	2.8
Sausage, pork	120	1.05	2.7
Sandwich meat	90	1.05	2.7
Cocoa powder	5	0.95	2.5
Butter	10	0.84	2.2
Margarine	10	0.84	2.2
Bread, brown	25	0.54	1.4
Bread, white	25	0.51	1.3

A.A. Paul and D.A.T. Southgate, *The Composition of Foods*, 1978.

Heart Association and World Health Organization both recommend a daily salt intake of 6 g per day. The American's salt consumption is now two to three times higher than the recommended intake.

What Types of Chronic Disease can be Caused by Consuming High-Salt Foods?

• Meta-analysis

Cardiovascular disease — People who consume high-salt foods have an increased risk of cardiovascular disease.

Twenty-five research papers evaluated the association between salt intake and cardiovascular disease in 274,683 people found that a daily intake of more than 12 g of salt per day increased the risk of cardiovascular disease by 12%. In brief, habitual consumption of high-salt foods could raise the risk of cardiovascular disease. Another meta-analysis of nineteen prospective studies examined the relationship between salt intake and cardiovascular disease including a total of 177,025 participants, of which 11,000 were cardiovascular disease cases. The results indicated that an increased intake of 5 g of salt per day raised the risk of cardiovascular disease by 17%.

Premature mortality — Frequent consumption of high-salt foods heightens the risk of premature mortality.

Twenty-five clinical studies on the association between salt intake and premature mortality in 274,683 people showed that high sodium intake of greater than 4.9 g per day increased the risk of all-cause mortality by 16%. In brief, daily consumption of high-salt foods greatly elevated the risk of premature mortality. Another meta-analysis of eleven prospective studies on the relationship between high-salt and premature mortality in 229,785 people revealed that high-sodium intake increased the risk of cardiovascular disease mortality by 12%.

Stomach cancer — Habitual consumption of high-salt foods can cause stomach cancer.

Seventy-six prospective studies investigated the effects of many dietary factors, including salt intake, on stomach cancer in a total of 6,316,385 subjects, of which 32,758 were gastric cancer cases. The results revealed that additional daily intake of 5 g of salt increased the risk of stomach cancer by 12%. In brief, a daily consumption of high-salt foods significantly elevated the risk of stomach cancer. Further supporting evidence about the harmful effects of high salt is presented in a meta-analysis of eleven clinical research reports in a total of 2,076,498 participants, of which 12,039 were gastric cancer cases, which showed that high salt consumption increased the risk of stomach cancer by 105%.

Stroke — People who regularly consume high-salt foods have a greater risk of stroke.

A meta-analysis of twelve epidemiological studies on the association between high-salt intake and stroke with 225,693 participants, of which 8,135 were stroke cases found that consumption of high-salt foods increase the risk of total stroke by 34%.

• Conclusion

In Table 36.2, the meta-analytical data has shown that consuming high-salt foods could lead to stroke, cardiovascular disease, stomach cancer, and even premature mortality. Consumption of high-salt foods increased the risk of stroke by 34% and the risk of cardiovascular disease by 12%. It is worth stressing that high consumption of salty foods increased the of stomach cancer by 105%. Furthermore, high salt consumption increased the risk of all-cause mortality and cardiovascular mortality by 16% and 12%, respectively.

In summary, high salt consumption is associated with an increased risk of stroke and cardiovascular disease. In addition,

Table 36.2. Meta-analytical Confirmation of High-salt Foods Associated with an Increased Risk of Chronic Diseases and Premature Mortality

Chronic Diseases	Increased Risk, High-salt Foods
Cardiovascular disease	Daily intake of more than 12 g of salt increased the risk of cardiovascular disease by 12%.
	Additional intake of 5 g of salt per day increased the risk of cardiovascular disease by 17%.
Premature mortality	Daily intake of more than 12.8 g of salt (4.9 g of sodium) increased the risk of all-cause mortality by 16%.
	High-salt diet increased the risk of all-cause mortality and cardiovascular disease mortality by 16% and 12%, respectively.
Stomach cancer	High-salt diet increased the risk of stomach cancer by 105%.
	Additional intake of 5 g of salt per day increased the risk of stomach cancer by 12%.
Stroke	High salt diet increased the risk of stroke by 34%.

regular high-salt intake can lead to stomach cancer. High-salt intake damages the cells lining the stomach wall, which causes ulcers and exacerbates the proliferation of *Helicobacter pylori*. The combination of stomach ulcers and the overgrowth of *Helicobacter pylori* can lead to stomach cancer.

• Recommendation

Prevention — People at risk of chronic disease should not consume more than 1 teaspoon of salt (or 6 g of salt) per day. Chronic disease patients should consume ½ teaspoon of salt (or 3–4 g of salt) per day.

Can eating too little salt also be harmful to health?

We have just talked about how eating too much salt is harmful to health. The question is, can eating too little salt be harmful to health as well? The answer is a resounding yes. Studies have shown that daily intake of salt less than 3 g may increase the risk of cardiovascular disease. In other words, too much salt intake increases the risk of cardiovascular disease, and too little salt intake can also increase the risk for cardiovascular disease. An extremely low sodium intake can trigger renin-aldosterone activity, stimulate sympathetic nervous system, lead to cardiovascular disease and elevate the risk of premature mortality. The symptoms of no salt intake include headache, nausea, vomiting, dizziness, confusion, and in severe cases brain edema. Hypertensive or other chronic diseases patients who have an extremely daily low salt intake may exacerbate the condition of their diseases. It is recommended that people should develop a healthy dietary habit of consuming one teaspoon of salt (6 g of salt) per day to maintain sodium-potassium balance and healthy metabolism in the body.

What Types of Chronic Disease can be Caused by No Salt Diet?

• Meta-analysis

Cardiovascular disease — Daily intake of extremely low-salt diet exacerbates the risk of cardiovascular disease.

A meta-analysis of 25 research articles examined the association between extremely low salt intake and cardiovascular disease in 274,683 people found that salt intake of less than 5 g per day increased the risk of cardiovascular disease by 10%.

Premature mortality — People who habitually consume extremely low-salt diet can heighten the risk of premature mortality.

Twenty-five clinical reports studied the relationship between low sodium intake and premature mortality revealed that low sodium intake of less than 2.6 g per day increased the risk of all-cause mortality by 9%.

• Conclusion

The meta-analytic data has revealed that habitual consumption of no salt or extremely low salt diet increased the risk of cardiovascular disease and premature mortality (see Table 36.3). Specifically, consumption of extremely low-salt diets increased the risk of cardiovascular disease by 10% and the risk of premature mortality by 9%. A no-salt diet does not equate to a healthy diet. Salt content in a healthy diet should not be less than 3 g per day; the ideal is preferably 6 g of salt per day.

In short, a no-salt diet can lead to cardiovascular disease and premature death.

Table 36.3.　Meta-analytical Confirmation of No-Salt Diet Associated with an Increased Risk of Cardiovascular Disease and Premature Mortality

Chronic Diseases	Increased Risk, No-Salt Diet
Cardiovascular disease	An extremely low-salt diet increased the risk of cardiovascular disease by 10%.
Premature mortality	An extremely low-salt diet increased the risk of all-cause mortality by 9%.

• Recommendation

Prevention — Everyone should not consume less than ½ teaspoon of salt (or 3–4 g of salt) per day.

37

Eggs

Early humans hunted and gathered eggs from oviparous animals. These oviparous animals included peacocks, pigeons, quail, plovers, partridges, sea gulls, wild turkeys, pelicans, wild geese and turtles, and the likes. Any eggs from oviparous animals were fair targets for early humans. In 6000 BCE, people in China harvested eggs from domesticated chickens. In the following millennia, chicken eggs became important and reliable food sources for peoples in the world.

Given suitable environment and conditions, an egg can hatch and become a chick. Eggs are packed with nutrients, including vitamins and essential elements, such as proteins, lipids, carbohydrates, calcium, magnesium, phosphorous, potassium, sodium, iron, zinc, Vitamin A, Vitamin D, Vitamin E, Vitamin K, and B vitamins, all of which are essential for the development and growth of newly hatched chicks.

How can egg consumption be harmful to health?

You may wonder: if chicken eggs were a reliable and dependable nutritious food for humans for thousands of years, why are we now concerned that egg consumption is harmful to health? The answer may have to do with the extension of the human lifespan. During the hunter-gatherer era, the average life expectancy of humans was only about 21–37 years and in 1900, the average American's life expectancy was only about 48 years. Currently, the average life expectancies of the American and the Japanese are about 78 and 82 years old, respectively. Chronic diseases, including heart disease, stroke, type 2 diabetes, and cognitive impairment, mainly occur at age 50 and older. The human's long-life expectancy allows the manifestation and onset of chronic disease at old ages. The life expectancy of early humans was very short. We probably will never find out whether egg consumption was harmful to early humans because they died at young ages. Consumption of eggs might be harmful to health for the following reasons.

- Fats — A mid-sized egg (44 g) contains about 5 g of animal fat. Eating two eggs is equal to an intake of 10 g of animal fats per day. High consumption of animal fat is known to increase the risk of cardiovascular disease and endometrial cancer.
- Cholesterol — A mid-sized egg (44 g) contains about 164 mg of cholesterol. Eating two eggs is equal to an intake of 328 mg of cholesterol per day. The American Heart Association recommends an upper intake limit of 300 mg cholesterol per day. Daily consumption of two eggs exceeds the upper intake limit of cholesterol.
- Choline — Egg yolk contains a high amount of choline, which is converted to trimethylamine-N-oxide by bacteria living in the gastrointestinal tract. High blood level of trimethylamine-N-oxide is linked to the higher risk of heart disease, stroke, and premature mortality.

In addition, egg consumption is linked to the risk of breast cancer and ovarian cancer, although the exact mechanism is not clear at present. One possible explanation is that eggs may contain environmental pollutants, organochlorine compounds, including dichlorodiphenyltrichloroethane (DDT) and hexachlorobenzene (HCB). These organochlorine compounds, which act as estrogens, may disrupt the female hormonal balance and increase the risk of breast cancer and ovarian cancer. In addition, polychlorinated biphenyls have been implicated in food contamination, including eggs. These carcinogenic organochlorine compounds can bind the aryl hydrocarbon receptor, negatively affect gene expression, and increase the risk of colorectal cancer.

What Types of Chronic Disease can be Caused by Egg Consumption?

• Meta-analysis

Breast cancer — Women who habitually consume eggs have a greater risk of breast cancer.

Thirteen research reports evaluated the relationship between egg intake and breast cancer found that consumption of 2–5 eggs per week increased the risk of breast cancer by 4%. Asian women who habitually consumed eggs increased the risk of breast cancer by 9%, while Western women who habitually consumed eggs increased the risk of breast cancer by 5%. In addition, postmenopausal women who regularly consumed eggs increased the risk of breast cancer by 6%.

Colorectal cancer — High egg consumption hastens the risk of colorectal cancer.

A meta-analysis of forty-four research articles studied the association between egg consumption and colorectal cancer in a total of 424,867 participants, of which 18,852 were colorectal cancer cases. The analysis showed that consumption of eggs increased the risk of colorectal cancer by 29%. Further analysis revealed that consumption of two eggs per week increased the risk of colorectal cancer by 14%, and consumption of more than two eggs per week increased the risk of colorectal cancer by 25%.

Heart disease — Habitual consumption of eggs exacerbates the risk of heart disease.

Four prospective cohorts explored the association between egg consumption and heart disease in a total of 105,999 subjects and 5,059 heart disease cases showed that consumption of eggs elevated the risk of heart failure by 25%. The dose-response studies revealed that consuming one or more eggs per day increased the risk of heart failure and coronary heart disease by 25% and 16%, respectively.

Ovarian cancer — Women who consume just one egg per day have a discernibly increased risk of ovarian cancer.

Twelve research reports on the relationship between egg consumption and ovarian cancer in a total of 629,453 participants including 3,728 ovarian cancer cases found that consumption of eggs increased the risk of ovarian cancer by 21%. In brief, women who consume eggs have an elevated risk of ovarian cancer. Additional supporting evidence about the harmful effects of eggs is documented in a meta-analysis, which showed that consumption of five eggs per week increased the risk of ovarian cancer by 9%.

Premature mortality — Daily consumption of eggs aggravates the risk of premature mortality.

Eight prospective studies on the association between egg consumption and premature mortality including 30,352 mortality cases revealed that egg consumption increased the risk of premature mortality by 6%. In addition, each additional intake of 50 g of eggs per day increased the risk of premature mortality by 15%.

Type 2 diabetes — People who consume more than two eggs per week have a greater risk of type 2 diabetes.

Fourteen prospective studies on the relationship between egg consumption and type 2 diabetes in 320,778 people found that the consumption of more than four eggs per week increased the risk of type 2 diabetes by 29% in pre-diabetic individuals. For type 2 diabetic patients, the consumption of more than four eggs per week increased the risk of cardiovascular disease by 40%. Analysis confirms that type 2 diabetic patients who consume eggs have an elevated risk of cardiovascular disease. Another meta-analysis of twelve research reports investigated the association between egg intake and type 2 diabetes included 287,963 participants, of which 16,264 were type 2 diabetes cases. The results showed that the consumption of more than two eggs per week increased the risk of type 2 diabetes by 18%, while consumption of one or two eggs per week did not seem to increase the risk of type 2 diabetes.

• Conclusion

As shown in Table 37.1, the meta-analytical results have demonstrated that egg consumption increased the risk of type 2 diabetes,

Table 37.1.   Meta-analytical Confirmation of Egg Consumption Associated with an Increased Risk of Chronic Diseases and Premature Mortality

Chronic Diseases	Increased Risk, Eggs
Breast cancer	Consumption of 2–5 eggs per week increased the risk of breast cancer by 4%.
	Eggs increased the risk of breast cancer in Asian women and Western women by 9% and 5%, respectively.
Colorectal cancer	Eggs increased the risk of colorectal cancer by 29%.
	Consumption of 2 eggs per week and more than 2 eggs per week increased the risk of colorectal cancer by 14% and 25%, respectively.
Heart disease	Egg consumption increased the risk of heart failure by 25%.
	One or more eggs daily increased the risk of heart failure and coronary heart disease by 25% and 16%, respectively.
Ovarian cancer	Eggs increased the risk of ovarian cancer by 21%.
	Women who consumed 5 eggs per week increased the risk of ovarian cancer by 9%.
Premature mortality	Eggs increased the risk of premature mortality by 6%.
	Each additional intake of 50 g of eggs per day increased the risk of all-cause mortality by 15%.
Type 2 diabetes	Consumption of more than 4 eggs per week increased the risk of type 2 diabetes by 29% in pre-diabetic individuals.
	Consumption of more than 4 eggs per week increased the risk of cardiovascular disease by 40% in patients with type 2 diabetes.

breast cancer, ovarian cancer, colorectal cancer, and premature mortality. Specifically, egg consumption has been found to increase the risk of type 2 diabetes by 29% and heart disease by 25%. Egg consumption also increased the risk of breast cancer by 9% and 5% in Asian women and Western women, respectively. In addition, consumption of eggs has been shown to increase the risk of ovarian cancer by 21%. The dose-response data revealed that consuming two eggs per week increased the risk of colorectal cancer by 14% and consuming more than two eggs per week increased the risk of colorectal cancer by 25%. Furthermore, egg consumption increased the risk of premature mortality by 6%.

- ## Recommendation

Prevention — People at risk of chronic diseases should not consume more than two eggs per week, and chronic disease patients should avoid consuming any egg.

Part Three

Twenty-one Chronic Diseases and Clinically Proven Antioxidant Foods

Most of the chronic diseases have complicated etiologies with modifiable and non-modifiable contributing factors. Non-modifiable factors, such as age, gender, family history, and genetics, cannot be controlled. However, modifiable factors include smoking, alcohol, lack of exercise, being overweight, and diet, which individuals can control. Studies maintain that diet alone could be responsible for at least one half of all chronic diseases.

Part Three reveals 21 chronic diseases and their corresponding clinically proven antioxidant foods as well as disease-causative foods, based on the meta-analytical results presented in Part One and Part Two. These chronic diseases are breast cancer, cardiovascular disease, chronic kidney disease, cognitive impairment, colorectal cancer, endometrial cancer, esophageal cancer, heart disease, hypercholesterolemia, hypertension, liver cancer, lung cancer, obesity, oral cancer, ovarian cancer, pancreatic cancer, premature mortality, prostate cancer, stomach cancer, stroke, and type 2 diabetes.

38

Breast Cancer

B reast cancer is a global public health issue. Every year, more than 1.7 million women are inflicted with the disease worldwide. In the United States, annually about 200,000 women and 2,000 men suffer from breast cancer. Over the years, the incident rate of breast cancer has been reduced in developed countries, while the incident rate of breast cancer is increasing in developing countries.

What types of antioxidant foods can prevent breast cancer?

Consumption of soy foods, fruits, vegetables, dairy foods, and dietary fiber lowered the risk of breast cancer in both pre- and post-menopausal women (see Table 38.1). Soy consumption reduced the risk of breast cancer by 32%. Intake of soy isoflavones reduced the risk of breast cancer by 41% in Asian women and by 8% in Western women. In addition, soy consumption reduced the risk of the breast cancer recurrence by 21%. Among fruits and vegetables, cruciferous vegetables, apples, and citrus fruits reduced the risk of breast cancer by 15%, 21%, and 10%, respectively. Moreover, milk and dietary fiber reduced the risk of breast cancer by 15% and 12%, respectively.

Table 38.1. Meta-analytical Confirmation of Antioxidant Foods for Breast Cancer

Antioxidant Foods	Reduced Risk, Breast Cancer
Dairy products	Dairy products reduced the risk of breast cancer by 15%. Among dairy products, low-fat milk, yogurt, and skim milk reduced the risk of breast cancer by 15%, 9%, and 10%, respectively.
Dietary fiber	Dietary fiber reduced the risk of breast cancer by 12%. Each additional intake of 10 g of dietary fiber reduced the risk of breast cancer by 4%.
Fruits	Fruits reduced the risk of breast cancer by 32%. Among fruits, citrus fruits and apples reduced the risk of breast cancer by 10% and 21%, respectively.
Soy foods	Soy foods reduced the risk of breast cancer by 32%. Soy foods reduced the risk of breast cancer recurrence by 21%. Intake of soy isoflavones reduced the risk of breast cancer in Asian women and Western women by 41% and 8%, respectively.
Vegetables	Vegetables reduced the risk of breast cancer by 23%. Among vegetables, cruciferous vegetables reduced the risk of breast cancer by 15%.

What types of harmful foods are linked to breast cancer?

As shown in Table 38.2, consumption of animal fats, red meat, processed meat, and eggs increased the risk of breast cancer in both pre- and postmenopausal women. High consumption of animal fats

Table 38.2. Meta-analytical Confirmation of Breast Cancer-causative Foods

Harmful Foods	Increased Risk, Breast Cancer
Animal fats	Animal fats increased the risk of breast cancer by 15%.
Eggs	Eggs increased the risk of breast cancer in Asian women and Western women by 9% and 5%, respectively. 2 to 5 eggs per week increased the risk of breast cancer by 4%. 9 eggs per week increased the risk of breast cancer by 9%.

Table 38.2. (*Continued*)

Harmful Foods	Increased Risk, Breast Cancer
Processed meat	Each additional intake of processed meat per day increased the risk of breast cancer by 9%.
Red meat	Each additional intake of red meat per day increased the risk of breast cancer by 13%.
Red meat and processed meat	Each additional intake of red meat and processed meat per day increased the risk of breast cancer by 7%.

increased the risk of breast cancer by 15%. Frequent consumption of red meat and processed meat increased the risk of breast cancer by 13% and 9%, respectively. Asian women who consumed eggs increased the risk of breast cancer by 9%, while Western women who consumed eggs increased the risk of breast cancer by 5%.

39

Cardiovascular Disease

Cardiovascular disease is a collective term for heart and vascular-related diseases, which include coronary heart disease and myocardial infarction. Cardiovascular disease is the leading cause of premature mortality worldwide. It is estimated that by 2030, about 23 million people in the world will die from cardiovascular disease. About 700,000 people die from cardiovascular disease each year in the US.

What types of antioxidant foods can prevent cardiovascular disease?

Consumption of tomatoes, berries, whole grain, tofu, low-fat milk, fruits, vegetables, olive oil, fish, and dietary fiber reduced the risk of cardiovascular disease (see Table 39.1). Tomato consumption decreased systolic blood pressure by 6 mmHg and the LDL cholesterol level by 4 mg/dL, both of which are risk factors of cardiovascular disease. Berry consumption decreased systolic blood pressure by 3 mmHg, LDL cholesterol level by 4 mg/dL, and fasting glucose level by 2 mg/dL, which are also contributing factors of cardiovascular disease. In addition, whole grains, fish, and low-fat milk reduced the risk of cardiovascular disease by 26%, 12%, and 12%, respectively. Cheese and tofu reduced the risk of cardiovascular disease by 18% and 20%, respectively.

Table 39.1. Meta-analytical Confirmation of Antioxidant Food Remedies for Cardiovascular Disease

Antioxidant Foods	Reduced Risk, Cardiovascular Disease
Berries	Berries decreased LDL cholesterol level by 3.8 mmHg and systolic pressure by 3 mmHg.
Dietary fiber	7 g of dietary fiber daily reduced the risk of cardiovascular disease by 9%.
Fish	2 to 4 servings of fish per week reduced the risk of cardiovascular disease by 6%. 5 or more servings of fish per week reduced the risk of cardiovascular disease by12%.
Fruits and vegetables	200 g of fruits and vegetables daily reduced the risk of cardiovascular disease by 8%. 800 g of fruits and vegetables daily reduced the risk of cardiovascular disease by 17%.
Olive oil	Olive oil reduced the risk of cardiovascular disease by 9%.
Tofu	Tofu reduced the risk of cardiovascular disease by 20%.
Tomatoes	Tomatoes decreased LDL cholesterol level by 4.0 mg/dL and systolic pressure by 5.7 mmHg.
Whole grains	45 g of whole grains daily reduced the risk of cardiovascular disease by 26%.

What types of harmful foods can cause cardiovascular disease?

As shown in Table 39.2, a high-salt diet increased the risk of cardiovascular disease by 12%, and a no-salt diet increased the risk of

Table 39.2. Meta-analytical Confirmation of Cardiovascular Disease-causative Foods

Harmful Foods	Increased Risk, Cardiovascular Disease
Extremely low salt	Less than 5 g of salt intake daily increased the risk of cardiovascular disease by 10%.
High salt	More than 12 g of salt intake daily increased the risk of cardiovascular disease by12%. Additional intake of 5 g of salt per day increased the risk of cardiovascular disease by 17%.

cardiovascular disease by 10%. Thus, neither high-salt diet nor no-salt diet is a healthy diet. In addition, an increased intake of 5 g of salt per day resulted in an increased risk of cardiovascular disease by 17%. Salt intake should be 6 g or 1 teaspoon per day to prevent the incidence of cardiovascular disease. Either too high or too little salt intake however can increase the risk of cardiovascular disease.

40

Chronic Kidney Disease

Chronic kidney disease is a condition manifested by a gradual loss of kidney functions. About 16.8% of all Americans aged 20 and older have chronic kidney disease. Severe chronic kidney disease can result in the total loss of kidney functions and require hemodialysis. A major challenge in the medical field is how to improve and maintain remaining kidney functions in patients with chronic kidney disease and prevent its progression to the end-stage renal failure.

What types of antioxidant foods can prevent chronic kidney disease?

Consumption of dietary fiber and soy food reduced inflammatory mediators as well as ameliorated the condition of the disease in patients with chronic kidney disease (see Table 40.1). Dietary fiber intake decreased serum uric acid level by 1.76 mmol/dL and

Table 40.1. Meta-analytical Confirmation of Antioxidant Food Remedies for Chronic Kidney Disease

Antioxidant Foods	Reduced risk, Chronic Kidney Disease
Dietary fibers	Foods rich in dietary fiber decreased serum uric acid level and serum creatinine level by 1.76 mmol/dL and 0.42 mg/dL, respectively.
Soy foods	Soy foods decreased serum creatinine level, serum phosphate, serum triglycerides, urine protein, and C-reactive protein by 0.05–0.11 mg/dL, 0.31 mg/dL, 4.1 mg/dL, 0.13 mg/day, and 0.98 mg/dL, respectively.

serum creatinine level by 0.42 mg/dL in chronic kidney disease patients. In addition, intake of soy protein decreased serum creatinine level by 0.05–0.11 mg/dL, serum triglycerides by 4.1 mg/dL, serum phosphate by 0.13 mg/dL, C-reactive protein by 0.98 mg/dL, and urine protein level by 0.13 mg/day in chronic kidney disease patients.

What types of harmful foods can cause chronic kidney disease?

Consumption of sugar-sweetened beverages has been shown to increase the risk of chronic kidney disease by 58% (see Table 40.2). The meta-analytical results are consistent with the view that habitual consumption of sugar-sweetened beverages can greatly increase the incidence of chronic kidney disease.

Table 40.2. Meta-analytical Confirmation of Chronic Kidney Disease-causative Foods

Harmful foods	Increased Risk, Chronic Kidney Disease
Sugar-sweetened beverages	Sugar-sweetened beverages increased the risk of chronic kidney disease by 58%.

41

Cognitive Impairment

Cognitive impairment is a neurological condition in which the gradual and progressive deterioration of memory, attention, and judgment negatively affect daily activities. In terms of the severity of the condition, cognitive impairment which is between normal aging and dementia is a dire global problem associated with population aging. Untreated, cognitive impairment can lead to dementia and even Alzheimer's disease. It is estimated that by the year 2050, globally, 14 million people will suffer from Alzheimer's disease.

What types of antioxidant foods can curtail cognitive impairment?

Regular consumption of fish, milk, fruits, and vegetables reduced the risk of cognitive impairment and dementia (see Table 41.1). Fish consumption reduced the risk of dementia by 20%. Each additional serving of fish per week reduced the risk of cognitive impairment by 5% and the risk of Alzheimer's disease by 7%. An intake of 4 ounces of fish per week reduced the risk of dementia by 12%. Milk consumption reduced the risk of cognitive impairment by 28%. Furthermore, each additional intake of 4 ounces of fruits and vegetables per day reduced the risk of cognitive impairment by 13%.

Table 41.1. Meta-analytical Confirmation of Antioxidant Food Remedies for Cognitive Impairment

Antioxidant Foods	Reduced Risk, Cognitive Impairment and Dementia
Fish	Each additional serving of fish per week reduced the risk of cognitive impairment by 5%.
	An intake of 4 ounces of fish per week reduced the risk of dementia by 12%
	Daily intake of 8 g of polyunsaturated fatty acids reduced the risk of cognitive impairment by 29%.
Fruits and vegetables	Fruits and vegetables reduced the risk of cognitive impairment by 37%.
	Each additional intake of 4 ounces of fruits and vegetables per day reduced the risk of cognitive impairment and dementia by 13%.
Milk	Milk intake reduced the risk of cognitive impairment by 28%.

42

Colorectal Cancer

Colorectal cancer is the second most common cancer in women and the third most common cancer in men. About 40% of Americans aged 60 and older have colon and/or rectal adenomas. Although most adenomas are benign and harmless, some adenomas may worsen and transform to colorectal cancer. Smoking, sedentary lifestyle, and unhealthy diet are the three major risk factors for colorectal cancer. In 2018, it is estimated that 97,220 new cases of colon cancer and 43,030 new cases of rectal cancer will be diagnosed, and 50,000 people will die from it in the United States.

What types of antioxidant foods can prevent colorectal cancer?

Nine food items, namely, fruits, vegetables, dietary fiber, soy foods, nuts, legumes, milk, whole grains, and fish reduced the risk of colorectal cancer. As shown in Table 42.1, fruits and vegetables reduced the risk of colorectal cancer by 18%. When analyzed separately, vegetables reduced the risk of colorectal cancer by 14%, while fruits reduced the risk of colorectal cancer by 15%. Further analysis revealed that broccoli and cruciferous vegetables reduced the risk of colorectal cancer by 20% and 16%, respectively. In addition, consumption of apples reduced the risk of colorectal cancer by 34%. Moreover, dietary fiber intake reduced the risk of colorectal cancer by 28%. When analyzed one at a time, whole grain dietary fiber, fruit dietary fiber, and vegetable dietary fiber reduced the risk of colorectal cancer by 17%, 7%, and 2%, respectively.

Table 42.1. Meta-analytical Confirmation of Antioxidant Food Remedies for Colorectal Cancer

Antioxidant Foods	Reduced Risk, Colorectal Cancer
Dietary fiber	Foods rich in dietary fiber reduced the risk of colorectal cancer by 28%. Each additional intake of 10 g of legume fiber, whole grain fiber, fruit fiber, and vegetable fiber reduced the risk of colorectal cancer by 38%, 17%, 7%, and 2%, respectively.
Fish	Fish reduced the risk of colorectal cancer by 7%.
Fruits	Fruits reduced the risk of colorectal cancer by 15%. Among fruits, apples reduced the risk of colorectal cancer by 34%.
Fruits and vegetables	Fruits and vegetables reduced the risk of colorectal cancer by 18%.
Legumes	Legumes reduced the risk of colorectal cancer by 18%.
Milk	Daily consumption of 200 ml of milk reduced the risk of colorectal cancer by 9%. Daily consumption of 525 ml of milk reduced the risk of colorectal cancer by 26% in men.
Nuts	Nuts reduced the risk of colorectal cancer by 24%
Soy foods	Soy foods reduced the risk of colorectal cancer by 21%.
Soy isoflavones	Soy isoflavones supplement reduced the risk of colorectal cancer by 24–30%. 20 mg of soy isoflavones daily reduced the risk of colorectal cancer by 8%.
Vegetables	Vegetables reduced the risk of colorectal cancer by 14%. Among the vegetables, cruciferous vegetables and broccoli reduced the risk of colorectal cancer by 16% and 20%, respectively.
Whole grains	Consumption of 90 g of whole grains per day reduced the risk of colorectal cancer by 17%.

Soy consumption reduced the risk of colorectal cancer by 21%, and consumption of foods rich in isoflavones reduced the risk of colorectal cancer by 24–30%. Furthermore, consumption of nuts, legumes, and whole grains reduced the risk of colorectal cancer by 24%, 18% and 17%, respectively. Finally, consumption of milk and fish reduced the risk of colorectal cancer by 9% and 7%, respectively.

What types of harmful foods are linked to colorectal cancer?

High consumption of red meat, processed meat, eggs, and high glycemic-load food increased the incidence of colorectal cancer (see Table 42.2). Consumption of four ounces of red meat per day increased the risk of colorectal adenomas by 27%, and consumption of two ounces of processed meat per day increased the risk of colorectal adenomas by 29%. When analyzed separately, beef consumption increased the risk of colorectal adenomas by 11%, while lamb consumption increased the risk of colorectal adenomas by 24%. In addition, habitual consumption of red meat increased the risk of colorectal cancer by 13%, and consumption of four ounces of red meat and processed meat per day increased the risk of colorectal cancer by 12%.

Moreover, habitual consumption of high glycemic-load foods such as white rice increased the risk of colorectal cancer by 26%. Lastly, high consumption of eggs increased the risk of colorectal cancer by 29%. Eating three eggs per week increased the risk of colorectal cancer by 14% and eating more than three eggs per week increased the risk of colorectal cancer by 25%.

Table 42.2.   **Meta-analytical Confirmation of Colorectal Cancer-causative Foods**

Harmful Foods	Increased Risk, Colorectal Cancer/Adenomas
Eggs	Eggs increased the risk of colorectal by 29%. 2 eggs per week increased the risk of colorectal cancer by 14%, and more than 2 eggs per week increased the risk of colorectal cancer by 25%.
High glycemic-load food	White rice increased the risk of colorectal cancer by 26%.
Processed meat	Each additional intake of 50 g of processed meat increased the risk of colorectal adenomas by 29%.
Red meat	Red meat increased the risk of colorectal cancer by 13%. Each additional intake of 100 g of red meat increased the risk of colorectal adenomas by 27%.
Red meat and processed meat	Red and processed meat increased the risk of colorectal cancer by 29%. Daily consumption of 4 ounces of red meat and processed meat increased the risk of colorectal cancer by 12%.

43

Endometrial Cancer

Endometrial cancer ranks as the fifth highest incident rate of gynecological cancers in developed countries. Each year, more than 600,000 women suffer from endometrial cancer in the United States. The two major risks for endometrial cancer are obesity and high blood estrogen level, both of which are associated, at least in part, with diets. Nutrient balance diet can control body weight, reduce blood estrogen level, and lower the risk of endometrial cancer.

What types of antioxidant foods can prevent endometrial cancer?

Frequent consumption of nuts, dietary fiber, soy foods, fruits, and vegetables can lower the risk of endometrial cancer in pre- and postmenopausal women, as shown in Table 43.1. Intake of nuts and dietary fiber reduced the risk of endometrial cancer by 42% and 30%, respectively. Soy consumption reduced the risk of endometrial cancer by 21% in Asian women and by 17% in Western women. Consumption of fruits and vegetables decreased the risk of endometrial cancer by 21%. When analyzed separately, consumption of cruciferous vegetables and fruits reduced the risk of endometrial cancer by 21% and 10%, respectively.

What types of harmful foods can cause endometrial cancer?

Consumption of high glycemic-load foods and foods rich in animal fat can significantly increase the risk of endometrial cancer in both

Table **43.1.** Meta-analytical Confirmation of Antioxidant Food Remedies for Endometrial Cancer

Antioxidant Foods	Reduced Risk, Endometrial Cancer
Dietary fiber	Foods rich in dietary fiber reduced the risk of endometrial cancer by 30%.
	Each additional intake of 5 g of dietary fiber per day reduced the risk of endometrial cancer by 18% in women on a daily 1,000-calorie diet.
Fruits	Fruits reduced the risk of endometrial cancer by 10%.
	Women who consumed 100 g of fruits per day reduced the risk of endometrial cancer by 3%.
Nuts	Tree nuts reduced the risk of endometrial cancer by 42%.
Soy foods	Soy foods reduced the risk of endometrial cancer in Asian women and Western women by 21% and 17%, respectively.
Vegetables	Vegetables reduced the risk of endometrial cancer by 21%. Among vegetables, cruciferous vegetables reduced the risk of endometrial cancer by 15%.
	Women who consumed 100 g of vegetables per day reduced the risk of endometrial cancer by 10%.

Table **43.2.** Meta-analytical Confirmation of Endometrial Cancer-causative Foods

Harmful Foods	Increased Risk, Endometrial Cancer
Animal fats	5 g and 10 g of animal fats daily increased the risk of endometrial cancer by 5% and 17%, respectively in women on a daily 1,000-calorie diet.
High glycemic-load foods	High glycemic-load foods increased the risk of endometrial cancer by 20%.
	High glycemic-load foods increased the risk of endometrial cancer by 54% in obese women.

pre- and postmenopausal women (see Table 43.2). Women who consumed high glycemic-load foods increased the risk of endometrial cancer by 28% and for obese women, consumption of high glycemic-load foods increased the risk of endometrial cancer by 54%. In addition, consumption of 5 g of animal fats increased the risk of endometrial cancer by 5% and consumption of 10 g of animal fats increased the risk of endometrial cancer by 17% in women on a daily 1,000-calorie diet.

44

Esophageal Cancer

Esophageal cancer is the eighth most common cancer. It is estimated that 500,000 people suffer from esophageal cancer worldwide and 38,000 people suffer from the cancer in the United States each year. The two major risk factors for esophageal cancer are smoking cigarettes and drinking alcohol. Alcohol can inhibit detox enzymes in the liver, result in the accumulation of carcinogenic compounds, and increase the risk of esophageal cancer. Carcinogenic compounds in cigarette smoke, such as lead, arsenic, benzene, nitrosamine, and polycyclic aromatic hydrocarbons, can cause damage to the DNA of the epithelial cells lining the esophagus, cause gene mutations, and increase the incidence of esophageal cancer.

What types of antioxidant foods can prevent esophageal cancer?

High consumption of dietary fiber, vegetables, fruits, and fish notably lowered the incident risk of esophageal cancer (see Table 44.1). Dietary fiber intake reduced the risk of esophageal cancer by 48%, and fruit and vegetable intake reduced the risk of esophageal cancer by 32%. When analyzed one by one, vegetable intake reduced the risk of esophageal cancer by 44%, and fruit intake reduced the risk of esophageal cancer by 47%. In addition, citrus fruit intake reduced the risk of esophageal cancer by 37%. Lastly, fish consumption reduced the risk of esophageal cancer by 9%.

Table 44.1. Meta-analytical Confirmation of Antioxidant Food Remedies for Esophageal Cancer

Antioxidant Foods	Reduced Risk, Esophageal Cancer
Citrus fruits	Citrus fruits reduced the risk of esophageal cancer by 37%.
Dietary fiber	Foods rich in dietary fiber reduced the risk of esophageal cancer by 48%. Each addition intake of 10 g of dietary fiber reduced the risk of esophageal cancer by 31%.
Fish	Fish intake reduced the risk of esophageal cancer by 9%.
Fruits	Fruits reduced the risk of esophageal cancer by 47%.
Fruits and vegetables	Fruits and vegetables reduced the risk of esophageal cancer by 32%.
Vegetables	Vegetables reduced the risk of esophageal cancer by 44%.

What types of harmful foods can cause esophageal cancer?

Frequent consumption of red meat and processed meat greatly increased the incidence of esophageal cancer (see Table 44.2). Consumption of red meat increased the risk of esophageal cancer by 42–55%, and consumption of processed meat increased the risk of esophageal cancer by 55%. Consumption of red meat and processed meat can greatly increase the incidence of esophageal cancer.

Table 44.2. Meta-analytical Confirmation of Esophageal Cancer-causative Foods

Harmful Foods	Increased Risk, Esophageal Cancer
Processed meat	Processed meat increased the risk of esophageal cancer by 55%.
Red meat	Red meat increased the risk of esophageal cancer by 42–55%. Daily intake of 120 g of red meat increased the risk of esophageal cancer by 35%.

45

Heart Disease

Heart disease has the highest mortality rate among all chronic diseases. In the United States, 600,000 people die from heart disease each year. Heart disease is caused in part by atherosclerosis, the hardening of blood vessels, due to high blood cholesterol or hypercholesterolemia, particularly high LDL cholesterol in the bloodstream. Inflammation causes leukocytes to release free radicals, which can oxidize LDL cholesterol to form oxidized LDL cholesterol. Oxidized LDL cholesterol is prone to stick on to the vessel wall and lead to atherosclerosis. Atherosclerotic lesions can form blood plagues, which narrow blood vessels and diminish blood flow. Ruptured blood plagues become blood clots, which flow into the heart via blood circulation and can result in heart disease, including heart attack and chest pain (angina).

What types of antioxidant foods can prevent heart disease?

Consumption of soy foods, nuts, fish, fruits, vegetables, legumes, and whole grains is associated with lower risks of heart disease (see Table 45.1). Soy foods reduced the risk of coronary heart disease by 34% and decreased triglycerides and LDL cholesterol levels by 10.7% and 5.5%, respectively, while they increased the HDL cholesterol level by 3.2%. Nut consumption reduced the risk of ischemic heart disease by 22%. In

Table 45.1. Meta-analytical Confirmation of Antioxidant Food Remedies for Heart Disease

Antioxidant Foods	Reduced Risk, Heart Disease
Fish	Fish intake of 1 serving, 2–4 servings, and more than 5 servings per week reduced the risk of heart disease by 9%, 13%, and 14%, respectively. 20 g of fish per week reduced the risk of heart failure by 6%.
Fruits and vegetables	Fruits and vegetables reduced by the risk of coronary heart disease by 17%.
Legumes	Legumes reduced the risk of ischemic heart disease by 14%.
Nuts	28.5 g of mixed nuts per week reduced the risk of ischemic heart disease by 22%.
Soy foods	Soy foods reduced the risk of coronary heart disease by 34%.

addition, fish consumption reduced the risk of acute coronary syndrome by 21%. Furthermore, fruits and vegetables reduced the risk of coronary heart disease by 17% and legumes reduced the risk of ischemic heart disease by 14%.

What types of harmful foods are linked to heart disease?

High consumption of red meat, processed meat, egg, and sugar-sweetened beverages greatly increased the risk of heart disease (see Table 45.2). Habitual consumption of processed meat, such as sausages, hotdogs, bacon, and ham, increased the risk of coronary heart disease by 42%. Consuming more than two eggs per week increased the risk of heart failure by 25%. In addition, sugar-sweetened beverages increased the risk of coronary heart disease by 16% and the risk of myocardial infarction by 19%.

Table 45.2. Meta-analytical Confirmation of Heart Disease-causative Foods

Harmful Foods	Increased Risk, Heart Disease
Eggs	Eggs increased the risk of heart failure by 25%.
	1 or more eggs daily increased the risk of heart failure and coronary heart disease by 25% and 16%, respectively.
Processed meat	Processed meat increased the risk of coronary heart disease and heart failure by 27% and 12%, respectively.
	Each additional intake of 50 g of processed meat per day increased the risk of coronary heart disease by 42%.
Red meat	Red meat increased the risk of coronary heart disease and heart failure by 15% and 8%, respectively.
Sugar-sweetened beverages	Sugar-sweetened beverages increased the risk of myocardial infarction by 19%.
	Each additional serving of sugar-sweetened beverages per day increased the risk of coronary heart disease by 16%.

46

Hypercholesterolemia (High Blood Cholesterol)

Hypercholesterolemia (high blood cholesterol), a condition characterized by high LDL cholesterol and high triglycerides, is the major risk factor for heart disease and stroke. About 73 million Americans have high LDL cholesterol levels (or "bad" cholesterol) and another 31 million have high total blood cholesterol levels. Cholesterol, a wax-like fatty substance, plays a multitude of important physiological roles, including the involvement in the production of sex hormones, Vitamin D, and gallbladder juice. Cholesterol in the cell membranes can modulate membrane fluidity and control the transport of substances across the cell membranes. Cholesterol is crucial for maintaining normal cellular functions and for supporting cardiovascular health. Most of the cholesterol however is produced in the body and only a small amount is derived from food intake.

What types of antioxidant foods can lower blood cholesterol?

Eleven food items favorably improved blood lipids and lipoproteins in patients with hypercholesterolemia. These eleven food items are avocados, cinnamon, garlic, whole grains, rice bran oil, legumes, cocoa/dark chocolate, nuts, soy foods, ginger, and cheese (see Table 46.1). Daily consumption of avocado decreased the total cholesterol level by 19 mg/dL, LDL cholesterol level by 17 mg/dL and triglycerides by 27 mg/dL in patients with hypercholesterolemia.

Table 46.1. Meta-analytical Confirmation of Antioxidant Food Remedies for Hypercholesterolemia

Antioxidant Foods	Reduced Risk, Hypercholesterolemia
Avocado	Avocado decreased total cholesterol level by 19 mg/dL, LDL cholesterol level by 17 mg/dL, and triglycerides by 27 mg/dL in hypercholesterolemic patients.
Cheese	Daily intake of 5 ounces of cheese reduced LDL cholesterol level by 6.5% and increased HDL cholesterol level by 3.5% in hypercholesterolemic patients.
Cinnamon	120 mg of cinnamon powder daily for 4–18 weeks reduced total cholesterol level by15.6 mg/dL, LDL cholesterol level by 9.42 mg/dL, and triglycerides by 30 mg/dL, as well as increased HDL cholesterol level by 1.66 mg/dL in hypertensive patients.
Cocoa products/ dark chocolate	Cocoa products/dark chocolate reduced total cholesterol level by 6.2 mg/dL and LDL cholesterol level by 5.9 mg/dL in hypercholesterolemic patients.
Garlic	Garlic power reduced total cholesterol level by 17.3 mg/dL and LDL cholesterol level by 8.1 mg/dL in hypercholesterolemic patients.
Ginger	Ginger decreased triglycerides by 1.6 mg/dL and increased HDL cholesterol level by 1.2 mg/dL in hypercholesterolemic patients.
Legumes	Legumes reduced total cholesterol level by 11.8 mg/dL and LDL cholesterol level by 8.0 mg/dL in hypercholesterolemic patients.
Nuts	60 g of nuts daily reduced total cholesterol level by 4.7 mg/dL, LDL cholesterol level by 4.8 mg/dL, and triglycerides by 2.2 mg/dL in hypercholesterolemic patients. 29–69 g of hazelnuts daily for 28 to 84 days reduced total cholesterol level by 2.3 mg/dL, LDL cholesterol level by 2.7 mg/dL in hypercholesterolemic patients. 43 g of almonds five times per week reduced total cholesterol level by 2.8 mg/dL, LDL cholesterol level by 2.2 mg/dL, and triglycerides by 1.2 mg/dL in hypercholesterolemic patients.
Rice bran oil	Rice bran oil decreased total cholesterol level by 13 mg/dL, LDL cholesterol level by 7 mg/dL, and increased HDL cholesterol level by 7 mg/dL in hypercholesterolemic patients.

Table 46.1. (*Continued*)

Antioxidant Foods	Reduced Risk, Hypercholesterolemia
Soy foods	Soy foods reduced total cholesterol level by 5.3 mg/dL, LDL cholesterol level by 4.8 mg/dL, and triglycerides by 4.9 mg/dL, and increased HDL cholesterol level by 1.4 mg/dL in hypercholesterolemic patients.
Soy proteins	25 g of soy proteins daily reduced total cholesterol level by 4.0 mg/dL, LDL cholesterol level by 4.2 mg/dL, and triglycerides by 1.5 mg/dL in hypercholesterolemic patients.
Whole grains	Whole grains reduced total cholesterol level by 15.1 mg/dL and LDL cholesterol level by 13.1 mg/dL in hypercholesterolemic patients.

The extent to which consumption of avocado decreases blood cholesterol levels resembles that observed by cholesterol lowering medications. Cinnamon powder intake decreased the total cholesterol level by 15.6 mg/dL, LDL cholesterol level by 9.42 mg/dL, and triglycerides by 30 mg/dL in patients with hypercholesterolemia. In addition, garlic consumption decreased the total cholesterol level by 17.3 mg/dL and LDL cholesterol level by 8.1 mg/dL, and increased the HDL cholesterol level by 2 mg/dL and whole grain consumption decreased the total cholesterol level by 15.1 mg/dL and LDL cholesterol level by 13.1 mg/dL.

Furthermore, consumption of rice bran oil decreased the total cholesterol level by 13 mg/dL, LDL cholesterol level by 7 mg/dL and increased the HDL cholesterol level by 7 mg/dL, while the consumption of cocoa/dark chocolate decreased the total cholesterol level by 6 mg/dL and LDL cholesterol level by 6 mg/dL. Nut consumption was also found to decrease the total cholesterol level by 5 mg/dL, LDL cholesterol level by 5 mg/dL and triglycerides by 2 mg/dL in hypercholesterolemic patients. Soy consumption, on the other hand, decreased the total cholesterol level by 5.3 mg/dL, LDL cholesterol level by 4.8 mg/dL, and increased the HDL cholesterol level by 1.4 mg/dL. Furthermore, ginger consumption decreased triglycerides by 1.6 mg/dL and increased the HDL cholesterol level by 1.2 mg/dL, and cheese consumption decreased the

Table 46.2. Meta-analytical Confirmation of Hypercholesterolemia-causative Foods

Harmful Foods	Increased Risk, Hypercholesterolemia
Fructose	100 g of fructose daily increased LDL cholesterol level by 11.6 mg/dL and triglycerides by 13.0 mg/dL.
Palm oil	Palm oil increased total cholesterol level by 6.4 mg/dL and LDL cholesterol level by 4.5 mg/dL.

LDL cholesterol level by 6.5% and increased the HDL cholesterol level by 3.5%.

What types of harmful foods can cause high blood cholesterol?

High consumption of fructose and palm oil can increase the total cholesterol level, LDL cholesterol level and triglycerides and heighten the risk of hypercholesterolemia, as shown in Table 46.2. Consumption of three cans of sugar-sweetened beverages daily increased the LDL cholesterol level by 11.6 mg/dL and triglycerides by 13.0 mg/dL, and consumption of palm oil raised the total cholesterol level by 6.4 mg/dL and the LDL cholesterol level by 4.5 mg/dL.

47

Hypertension

Globally, 1.2 billion people suffer from hypertension, a chronic disease that has now become a major health problem worldwide. The incident rate of hypertension is related to the socioeconomic condition of the country — the higher the per capita income of the country, the lower the incident rate of hypertension and the opposite is true. To date, South Asia and Africa have the highest incident rates of hypertension. Complications from hypertension include stroke, heart disease, and kidney disease, which result in 80 million deaths per year, or about 13% of all mortalities in the world. Hypertension is defined as systolic pressure equal to or higher than 140 mmHg and diastolic pressure equal to or higher than 90 mmHg. The early stage of hypertension is often symptomless. About 75 million people in the United States suffer from hypertension, which is about one third of adult population. Every day, 1,000 people die from hypertension and its complications in the United States alone.

What types of antioxidant foods can lower blood pressure?

Table 47.1 illustrates 11 meta-analytically identified anti-hypertensive food items. These food items are resveratrol, garlic, low salt, grape seed extract, soy foods, fruits, vegetables, low-fat milk, flaxseeds, dietary fiber, pomegranates, and nuts. Among these food items, resveratrol appears to be most effective in lowering blood pressure in both pre-hypertensive individuals and hypertensive

Table 47.1. Meta-analytical Confirmation of Antioxidant Food Remedies for Hypertension

Antioxidant Foods	Reduced Risk, Hypertension
Dietary fiber	Dietary fiber reduced systolic pressure by 0.9 mmHg and diastolic pressure by 0.7 mmHg in hypertensive patients.
Flaxseeds	Flaxseed extract reduced systolic pressure by 2.9 mmHg and diastolic pressure by 2.4 mmHg in hypertensive patients. Whole flaxseeds decreased diastolic pressure by 2 mmHg in hypertensive patients.
Fruits	Fruits reduced the risk of hypertension by 13%.
Fruits and vegetables	Fruits and vegetables reduced the risk of hypertension by 10%.
Garlic	Garlic reduced systolic pressure by 8.7 mmHg and diastolic pressure by 6.1 mmHg in hypertensive patients. Garlic reduced systolic pressure by 5.1 mmHg and diastolic pressure by 2.5 mmHg in pre-hypertensive patients.
Grape seed extract	Grape seed extract reduced systolic pressure by 6.1 mmHg and diastolic pressure by 2.8 mmHg in hypertensive patients. Grape seed extract reduced systolic pressure by 6.0 mmHg and diastolic pressure by 3.1 in middle-age hypertensive patients. Grape seed extract decreased systolic pressure by 8.5 mmHg in hypertensive patients with metabolic syndrome.
Low-fat milk	200 ml of low-fat milk daily reduced the risk of hypertension by 4%.
Low salt	6 g of salt daily reduced systolic pressure by 3.5 mmHg and diastolic pressure by 1.5 mmHg in hypertensive patients. 4.4 g of salt daily for 4 weeks reduced systolic pressure by 4.2 mmHg and diastolic pressure by 2.1 mmHg in pre-hypertensive individuals. 4.4 g of salt daily for four weeks reduced systolic pressure by 5.4 mmHg and diastolic pressure by 2.8 mmHg in hypertensive patients.
Milk proteins	Milk proteins decreased systolic pressure by 3.3 mmHg and diastolic pressure by 1.1 mmHg in hypertensive patients.
Nuts	Nuts reduced the risk of hypertension by 8% in pre-hypertensive individuals.
Pistachios	Pistachios reduced systolic pressure by 1.8 mmHg and diastolic pressure by 0.8 mmHg in pre-hypertensive individuals.

Table 47.1. (*Continued*)

Antioxidant Foods	Reduced Risk, Hypertension
Pomegranates	240 ml of pomegranate juice daily reduced systolic pressure by 5.0 mmHg and diastolic pressure by 2.0 mmHg in hypertensive patients.
	Daily consumption of 100–200 ml of pomegranate juice decreased systolic pressure by 11.0 mmHg and diastolic pressure by 4 mmHg in hypertensive patients.
Resveratrol	150 mg of resveratrol daily reduced systolic pressure by 11.9 mmHg in hypertensive patients.
Soy foods	Soy foods decreased systolic pressure by 2.5 mmHg and diastolic pressure by 1.5 mmHg in pre-hypertensive individuals.
	Soy foods decreased systolic pressure by 5.9 mmHg and diastolic pressure by 3.4 mmHg in hypertensive patients.
Vegetables	Vegetables reduced the risk of hypertension by 12%

patients. Intake of resveratrol has been found to reduce systolic pressure by 11.9 mmHg in hypertensive patients. The extent to which blood pressure reduced by resveratrol is like the reduction observed by anti-hypertension medications. The major difference between resveratrol and anti-hypertension medications is that the former is natural with no known side-effects, while the latter are synthetic with potential side-effects and additional costs.

Garlic intake has been shown to decrease systolic pressure by 8.7 mmHg and diastolic pressure by 6 mmHg in hypertensive patients. A daily consumption of pomegranate juice (100–200 ml) decreased systolic pressure by 11.0 mmHg and diastolic pressure by 4 mmHg in hypertensive patients. Intake of grape seed extract decreased systolic pressure by 6.1 mmHg and diastolic pressure by 2.8 mmHg, and soy consumption decreased systolic pressure by 2.5 mmHg and diastolic pressure by 1.5 mmHg in hypertensive patients. Moreover, flaxseeds decreased systolic pressure by 2.9 mmHg and diastolic pressure by 2.4 mmHg in hypertensive patients.

Table 47.2.   Meta-analysis Confirmation of Hypertension-causative Foods

Harmful Foods	Increased Risk, Hypertension
Artificially-sweetened beverages	Artificially-sweetened beverages increased the risk of hypertension by 15%.
Sugar-sweetened beverages	Sugar-sweetened beverages increased the risk of hypertension by 12%. Each additional serving of sugar-sweetened beverages per day increased the risk of hypertension by 8%.

In addition, fruits and vegetables reduced the risk of hypertension by 10%. When analyzed separately, fruits reduced the risk of hypertension by 13%, while vegetables reduced the risk of hypertension by 12%. Finally, nuts and low-fat milk reduced the risk of hypertension by 8% and 4%, respectively.

What types of harmful foods are linked to high blood pressure?

High consumption of sugar-sweetened beverages and artificially-sweetened beverages exacerbated the risk of hypertension (see Table 47.2). High consumption of sugar-sweetened beverages and artificially-sweetened beverages heightened the risk of hypertension by 12% and 15%, respectively.

48

Liver Cancer

L iver cancer has the second highest mortality rate among all human cancers and globally, 780,000 people die from liver cancer each year. The major risk factors for liver cancer are hepatitis B and hepatitis C infections, smoking cigarettes, and alcohol consumption. In the United States, 40,000 people suffer from liver cancer each year.

What types of antioxidant foods can prevent liver cancer?

Consumption of fish and vegetable lowered the risk of liver cancer (see Table 48.1). Habitual consumption of n-3 polyunsaturated fatty acids reduced the risk of liver cancer by 51%, whereas habitual consumption of fish reduced the risk of liver cancer by 29%. In addition, a daily intake of 100 g of vegetables reduced the risk of liver cancer by 8%.

Table 48.1.   Meta-analytical Confirmation of Antioxidant Food Remedies for Liver Cancer

Antioxidant Foods	Reduced Risk, Liver Cancer
Fish	Fish intake reduced the risk of liver cancer by 29%.
Vegetables	Vegetables reduced the risk of liver cancer by 28%. Each additional intake of 100 g of vegetables per day reduced the risk of liver cancer by 8%.

49

Lung Cancer

Lung cancer is the second most common cancer in the United States, and it has the highest mortality rate in women among all cancers worldwide. Smoking and second-hand smoking are the two major risk factors for lung cancer. Cooking fumes and indoor pollution can also raise the incident rate of lung cancer. One of every 15 houses in the United States emits radioactive radon gas from the indoor walls. Long-term exposure to radon gas can heighten the incident risk of lung cancer, and indoor radon gas becomes the second major risk factor of lung cancer. About 220,000 people suffer from lung cancer each year in the United States.

What types of antioxidant foods can prevent lung cancer?

Consumption of soy foods, fruits, vegetables, and fish lowered the risk of lung cancer as shown in Table 49.1. Women who consumed soy foods reduced the risk of lung cancer by 37%, while female non-smokers who consumed soy foods reduced the risk of lung cancer by 41%. In addition, soy isoflavones reduced the risk of lung cancer by 24%. Moreover, fruits and vegetables reduced the risk of lung cancer by 14%. When analyzed one at a time, vegetables reduced the risk of lung cancer by 8%, and fruits reduced the risk of lung cancer by 18%. The does-response studies have shown that each additional intake of 100 g of fruits per day reduced the risk of lung cancer by 8%, and each additional intake of 100 g of vegetables per day reduced the risk of lung cancer by 6%. When analyzed

Table 49.1. Meta-analytical Confirmation of Antioxidant Food Remedies for Lung Cancer

Antioxidant Foods	Reduced Risk, Lung Cancer
Cruciferous vegetables	Women who consumed cruciferous vegetables reduced the risk of lung cancer by 27%, and non-smoking women who consumed cruciferous vegetables reduced the risk of lung cancer by 41%.
Fish	Fish intake reduced the risk of lung cancer by 21%.
Fruits	Fruits reduced the risk of lung cancer by 18%. Each additional intake of 100 g of fruits per day reduced the risk of lung cancer by 15%.
Fruits and vegetables	Fruits and vegetables reduced the risk of lung cancer by 14%.
Soy foods	Soy foods reduced the risk of lung cancer by 29%. Soy foods reduced the risk of lung cancer in women and non-smoking women by 37% and 41%, respectively.
Vegetables	Vegetables reduced the risk of lung cancer by 9%. Each additional intake of 100 g of vegetables per day reduced the risk of lung cancer by 18%.

one by one, a daily intake of 1½ cups of vegetables reduced the risk of lung cancer by 6%, while a daily intake of 1½ cups of fruits reduced the risk of lung cancer by 8%. A daily intake of five cups of fruits and vegetables provided the best protection against the incidence of lung cancer. Furthermore, cruciferous vegetables and apples reduced the risk of lung cancer by 27% and 25%, respectively. Last, but not least, fish consumption reduced the risk of lung cancer by 21%.

What types of harmful foods can cause lung cancer?

Habitual consumption of red meat and processed meat can elevate the risk of lung cancer as shown in Table 49.2. A daily consumption of a piece of 4-ounce steak increased the risk of the incidence of lung cancer by 35%, and a daily consumption of 2 pieces of bacon or 1 hotdog increased the risk of the incidence of lung cancer by 20%.

Table 49.2.   Meta-analytical Confirmation of Lung Cancer-causative Foods

Harmful Foods	Increased Risk, Lung Cancer
Processed meat	Processed meat increased the risk of lung cancer by 23%. Each additional intake of 50 g of processed meat per day increased the risk of lung cancer by 20%.
Red meat	Red meat increased the risk of lung cancer by 44%. Each additional intake of 120 g of red meat per day increased the risk of lung cancer by 35%.

50

Obesity

Obesity is a chronic disease in which the body stores excessive amounts of fats to the extent that becomes harmful to health. Overeating, a sedentary lifestyle, and genetics can lead to excessive fat storage in the body. Obesity is the risk factor for many other chronic diseases, including heart disease, stroke, and type 2 diabetes. About one-half of the adult population in the United States are overweight and one-third are obese. In other words, 150 million people are overweight, and another 100 million people are obese in the United States. In 2016, more than 124 million of children and teenagers are obese in the world, compared to only 11 million of children and teenagers in 1975, according to the data from World Health Organization. During the past forty years, there has been a 10-fold increase in the number of obese children and teenagers worldwide.

The bookstores are chock full of all kinds of diet-related books. Basically, if you follow the dietary advice provided in those diet books, you will lose some weight. However, when the specified diet program time expired, often, you will regain your lost weight. This is neither a diet book nor a recipe book. In this chapter, we focus on a list of meta-analytical identified food items, including fruits, vegetables, legumes, dairy foods, and whole grains, that have been shown to exhibit anti-obesity properties. Eating the right kinds of foods instead of counting calories is the best way for weight loss.

What types of antioxidant foods can lower body weight?

Regular consumption of fruits, vegetables, dairy foods, legumes, and whole grains was found to be effective in reducing body weight in overweight and obese individuals as shown in Table 50.1. Regular consumption of blueberries and apples/pears reduced 1.11 and 1.24 lbs in body weight in overweight and obese individuals, respectively. In addition, consumption of soy foods and cruciferous vegetables reduced 2.47 and 1.37 lbs in overweight and obese individuals, respectively. Furthermore, dairy foods, such as milk, reduced the risk of obesity by 47% in children and the risk of obesity by 25% in adults. Lastly, consumption of legumes and whole grains reduced 0.8 and 0.8 lb. in body weight, respectively.

Table 50.1. Meta-analytical Confirmation of Antioxidant Food Remedies for Obesity

Antioxidant Foods	Reduced Risk, Obesity
Apples	Each additional serving of apples per day reduced 1.2 lbs in weight.
Blueberries	Each additional serving of blue berries per day reduced 1.11 lb in weight.
Cruciferous vegetables	Each additional serving of cruciferous vegetables per day reduced 1.37 lbs in weight.
Dairy foods	Dairy foods daily reduced the risk of obesity in children and adults by 46% and 25%, respectively. Daily intake of milk reduced the risk of obesity in children and adults by 17% and 23%, respectively. Each additional intake of 200 ml of milk per day decreased the risk of obesity by 16%.
Legumes	Legumes reduced 0.75 lb in weight.
Soy foods	Each additional serving of soy foods per day reduced 2.47 lb in weight.
Whole grains	48–80 g of whole grains daily reduced 0.8 lb in weight.

What types of harmful foods can cause weight gain?

Habitual consumption of sugar-sweetened beverages increased 1.9 lbs in body weight. In addition, high consumption of sugar-sweetened beverages increased the risk of obesity by 18%, while high consumption of artificially sweetened beverages increased the risk of obesity by 59% (see Table 50.2).

Table 50.2.   Meta-analytical Confirmation of Obesity-causative Foods

Harmful Foods	Increased Risk, Obesity
Artificially sweetened beverages	Artificially-sweetened beverages increased the risk of obesity by 59%.
Sugar-sweetened beverages	Sugar-sweetened beverages increased weight gain by 1.9 lb and increased the risk of obesity by 18%.
	Each additional intake of one can of sugar-sweetened beverages per day increased weight gain by 0.5 lb.

51

Oral Cancer

The oral cavity is the area where we taste and chew our food. Globally, about 450,000 people suffer from oral cancer each year, and in the United States, about 50,000 people are inflicted with oral cancer. The five-year survival rate of oral cancer is about 50%. The three major risk factors for oral cancer are chewing areca nut, smoking cigarettes, and drinking alcohol.

What types of foods can prevent oral cancer?

Consumption of fruits and vegetables greatly decreased the incidence of oral cancer, as shown in Table 51.1. People who habitually consumed fruits and vegetables reduced the risk of oral cancer by 46%. The dose-response analysis has shown that each additional serving of fruits per day reduced the risk of oral cancer by 49%, and each additional serving of vegetables per day reduced the risk of oral cancer by 50%.

Table 51.1. Meta-analytical Confirmation of Antioxidant Food Remedies for Oral Cancer

Antioxidant Foods	Reduced Risk, Oral Cancer
Fruits	Each additional serving of fruits by per day reduced the risk oral cancer by 49%.
Fruits and vegetables	Fruits and vegetables reduced the risk of oral cancer by 46%.
Vegetables	Each additional serving of vegetables per day reduced the risk of oral cancer by 50%.

What types of harmful foods are linked to oral cancer?

Chewing areca nuts and consumption of red and processed meat
heightened the risk of oral cancer (see Table 51.2). The Taiwanese
who chewed areca nuts had a 7-fold increase in the incident rate of
oral cancer. In addition, people who chewed areca nuts and smoked
cigarettes had a 6.5-fold increase in the risk of oral cancer, whereas
people who chewed areca nuts, smoked cigarette, and consumed
alcohol beverages had a 39-fold increase in the risk of oral cancer.
Finally, consumption of processed meat increased 91% risk of oral
cancer.

Table 51.2.   Meta-analytical Confirmation of Oral Cancer-causative Foods

Harmful Foods	Increased Risk, Oral Cancer
Areca nuts	Chewing areca nuts increased the risk of oral cancer 5.2-fold.
	Chewing areca nuts and smoking cigarettes increased the risk of oral cancer 6.5-fold.
	Chewing areca nuts, smoking cigarettes, and drinking alcohol increased the risk of oral cancer 39-fold.
Processed meat	Processed meat increased the risk of oral cancer by 91%.
Red meat	Red meat increased the risk of oral cancer by 5%.
Red meat and processed meat	Red meat and processed meat increased the risk of oral cancer by 14%.

52

Ovarian Cancer

Globally, about 200,000 women suffer from ovarian cancer each year, according to the data from the World Health Organization. Ovarian cancer is the sixth most common cancer among all gynecological cancers. Although the incident rate of ovarian cancer is low compared to that of breast cancer or endometrial cancer, it has the highest mortality rate. Once diagnosed, there is a 70% chance that the cancer might have already spread to other parts of the body. The 5-year survival rate of ovarian cancer is only about 20–30%. Obesity is the major risk factor of ovarian cancer. Currently, about 35% of all adult women are obese in the United States.

What types of antioxidant foods can prevent ovarian cancer?

Frequent consumption of soy foods and cruciferous vegetables lowered the risk of ovarian cancer in both pre- and postmenopausal women as shown in Table 52.1. Women who consumed soy foods

Table 52.1. Meta-analytical Confirmation of Antioxidant Food Remedies for Ovarian Cancer

Antioxidant Foods	Reduced Risk, Ovarian Cancer
Cruciferous vegetables	Cruciferous vegetables reduced the risk of ovarian cancer by 14%.
Soy foods	Soy foods reduced the risk of ovarian cancer by 39%.
Soy isoflavones	Soy isoflavone supplement reduced the risk of ovarian cancer by 30%.

and cruciferous vegetables reduced the risk of ovarian cancer by 39% and 14%, respectively. Cruciferous vegetables include broccoli, cauliflower, and cabbage, and soy foods include tofu, soybean, and soy milk.

What types of harmful foods can cause ovarian cancer?

High consumption of animal fats and eggs greatly elevated the risk of ovarian cancer (see Table 52.2). Consumption of foods high in animal fat increased the risk of ovarian cancer by 70%, and consumption of foods high in saturated fat increased the risk of ovarian cancer by 24%. In addition, egg consumption increased the risk of ovarian cancer by 21%.

Table 52.2. Meta-analytical Confirmation of Ovarian Cancer-causative Foods

Harmful Foods	Increased Risk, Ovarian Cancer
Animal fats	High animal fats increased the risk of ovarian cancer by 70%.
Eggs	Eggs increased the risk of ovarian cancer by 21%. Women who consumed 5 eggs per week increased the risk of ovarian cancer by 9%.
Saturated fats	High saturated fat foods increased the risk of ovarian cancer by 24%.

53

Pancreatic Cancer

Pancreatic cancer ranks the fourth highest mortality rate among all cancers in the United States. About 300,000 people die from pancreatic cancer each year worldwide, and about 20,000 people die from pancreatic cancer in the United States. Smoking cigarettes, drinking alcoholic beverages, obesity, and type 2 diabetes are the major risk factors for pancreatic cancer.

What types of antioxidant foods can prevent pancreatic cancer?

Table 53.1 shows that consumption of dietary fiber, vegetables, fruits, whole grains, and nuts can reduce the risk of pancreatic

Table 53.1. Meta-analytical Confirmation of Antioxidant Food Remedies for Pancreatic Cancer

Antioxidant Foods	Reduced Risk, Pancreatic Cancer
Dietary fiber	Foods rich in dietary fiber reduced the risk of pancreatic cancer by 48%. Each additional intake of 10 g dietary fiber per day reduced the risk of pancreatic cancer by 12%.
Fruits	Fruits reduced the risk of pancreatic cancer by 29%.
Nuts	Nuts reduced the risk of pancreatic cancer by 32%.
Vegetables	Vegetables reduced the risk of pancreatic cancer by 38%.
Whole grains	Whole grains reduced the risk of pancreatic cancer by 24%. Whole grains reduced the risk of pancreatic cancer in Americans and Europeans by 36% and 5%, respectively.

cancer. Dietary fiber intake reduced the risk of pancreatic cancer by 48%, and each additional intake of 10 g of dietary fiber per day reduced the risk of pancreatic cancer by 12%. In addition, vegetable consumption reduced the risk of pancreatic cancer by 38%, while cruciferous vegetable consumption reduced the risk of pancreatic cancer by 22%. Furthermore, fruit consumption reduced the risk of pancreatic cancer by 29%, while citrus fruit consumption reduced the risk of pancreatic cancer by 17%. Moreover, whole grains reduced the risk of pancreatic cancer by 36% and 5% in Americans and Europeans, respectively. Finally, nut consumption reduced the risk of pancreatic cancer by 32%.

What types of harmful foods are linked to pancreatic cancer?

Red meat and processed meat consumption greatly augmented the risk of pancreatic cancer (see Table 53.2). A daily consumption of a piece of 4 ounces of steak can increase the risk of pancreatic cancer by 13%, and a daily consumption of two pieces of bacon or one hotdog can heighten the risk of pancreatic cancer by 19%.

Table 53.2.   Meta-analytical Confirmation of Pancreatic Cancer-causative Foods

Harmful Foods	Increased Risk, Pancreatic Cancer
Processed meat	Each additional intake of 50 g of processed meat per day increased the risk of pancreatic cancer by 19%.
Red meat	Red meat increased the risk of pancreatic cancer by 48%. Each additional intake of 120 g of red meat per day increased the risk of pancreatic cancer by 13%.

54

Premature Mortality

Premature mortality or early death refers to a situation in which the lifespan of a person is shorter than average life expectancy of the country in which he resides. For instance, currently, the average life expectancy of Americans is about 78 years. If an American died at age 68, he would have died prematurely by 10 years. The major risk factors for premature mortality include chronic diseases, such as hypertension, heart disease, stroke, type 2 diabetes, and cancers. Foods that reduce the risk of chronic diseases can prevent the incidence of premature mortality.

What types of antioxidant foods can prevent premature mortality?

Regular consumption of nuts, whole grains, dietary fiber, fruits, vegetables, and fish reduced the risk of premature mortality, as shown in Table 54.1. 10 g of mixed nuts daily reduced the risk of all-cause mortality, cardiovascular disease mortality, and neurodegenerative disease mortality by 27%, 39%, and 44%, respectively. In addition, nut consumption also reduced the risk of cancer mortality, infectious disease mortality, and kidney disease mortality by 15%, 75%, and 73%, respectively. Consumption of whole grain reduced the risk of all-cause mortality, cancer mortality, and diabetes mortality by 22%, 18%, and 51%, respectively. Moreover, consumption of whole grain also reduced risk of the risk of infectious disease mortality, cardiovascular disease mortality, and myocardial infarction mortality by 26%, 30%, and 32%, respectively.

Table 54.1. Meta-analytical Confirmation of Antioxidant Food Remedies for Preventing Premature Mortality

Antioxidant Foods	Risk Reduced, Premature Mortality
Dietary fiber	10 g of dietary fiber daily reduced the risk of all-cause mortality, cardiovascular mortality, coronary heart disease mortality, myocardial infarction mortality, and cancer mortality by 11%, 9%, 11%, 34%, and 6%, respectively.
Fish	Each additional intake of 15 g of fish per day reduced the risk of coronary heart disease by 6%. 60 g of fish daily reduced the risk of all-cause mortality by 12%.
Fruits and vegetables	200 g of fruits and vegetables daily reduced the risk of all-cause mortality, coronary heart disease mortality, stroke mortality, cardiovascular disease mortality, and cancer mortality by 10%, 8%, 16%, 8%, and 3%, respectively. Fruits and vegetables reduced the risk of breast cancer mortality by 8%. Separately, fruits reduced the risk of breast cancer mortality by 13% and vegetables reduced the risk of breast cancer mortality by 4%.
Nuts	1 serving of nuts per week reduced the risk of all-cause mortality by 4% and the risk of cardiovascular disease by 7%. 10 g of mixed nuts daily reduced the risk of all-cause mortality, neurodegenerative disease mortality, cardiovascular disease mortality, cancer mortality, and respiratory disease mortality by 27%, 44%, 17%, 15%, and 29%, respectively. 28 g of mixed nuts daily reduced the risk of all-cause mortality, respiratory disease mortality, type 2 diabetes mortality, neurodegenerative disease mortality, infectious disease mortality, and kidney disease mortality by 28%, 52%, 23%, 35%, 75%, and 73%, respectively.
Whole grains	50 g of whole grains daily reduced the risk of all-cause mortality, cardiovascular disease mortality, myocardial infarction mortality, and cancer mortality by 22%, 30%, 32%, and 18%, respectively. 90 g of whole grains daily reduced the risk of all-cause mortality, cancer mortality, respiratory disease mortality, diabetes mortality, and infectious disease mortality by 17%, 15%, 22%, 51%, and 26%, respectively.

Additionally, daily intake of 10 g of dietary fiber reduced the risk of all-cause mortality, cardiovascular disease mortality, coronary heart disease mortality, myocardial infarction mortality and cancer mortality by 11%, 9%, 11%, 34% and 6%, respectively.' Moreover, consumption of fruits and vegetables reduced the risk of all-cause mortality, coronary heart disease mortality, stroke mortality by 10%, 8%, and 16%, respectively. When analyzed separately, consumption of fruits reduced the risk of all-cause mortality by 9%, while consumption of vegetables reduced the risk of all-cause mortality by 7%. Lastly, fish consumption reduced the risk of all-cause mortality by 9% and the risk of coronary heart disease mortality by 6%.

What types of harmful foods can cause premature mortality?

High consumption of high salt/or salt, processed meat, red meat, and eggs increased the risk of premature mortality (see Table 54.2).

Table 54.2.   Meta-analytical Confirmation of Premature Mortality-causative Foods

Harmful Foods	Increased Risk, Premature Mortality
Eggs	Eggs increased the risk of premature mortality by 6%. Each additional intake of 50 g of eggs per day increased the risk of premature mortality by 15%.
Extremely low salt	Daily intake of less than 2.6 g of sodium per day increased the risk of all-cause mortality by 9%.
High salt	High-salt food increased the risk of all-cause mortality and cardiovascular disease mortality by 16% and 12%, respectively. Daily intake of more than 12.8 g of salt (4.9 g of sodium) per day increased the risk of all-cause mortality by 16%.
Processed meat	Each additional intake of 50 g of processed meat increased the risk of all-cause mortality by 23%. Each additional serving of processed meat per day increased the risk of all-cause mortality, cardiovascular mortality, and cancer mortality by 15%, 15%, and 8%, respectively.
Red meat	Red meat consumption increased the risk of all-cause mortality 10% and cardiovascular disease mortality by 16%. Each additional intake of 100 g of red meat increased the risk of all-cause mortality by 10%.
Red meat and processed meat	Red meat and processed meat increased the risk of all-cause mortality by 29%.

High sodium intake increased the risk of all-cause mortality by 16% and the risk of cardiovascular disease mortality by 12%. On the other hand, low sodium intake increased the risk of all-cause mortality by 9%. A no-salt diet is not a healthy diet. In addition, consumption of red meat increased the risk of all-cause mortality by 10% and the risk of cardiovascular disease mortality by 16%. While consumption of processed meat increased the risk of all-cause mortality, cardiovascular disease mortality, and cancer mortality by 23%, 18%, and 8%, respectively. Finally, high consumption of eggs increased the risk of premature mortality by 11%.

55

Prostate Cancer

Prostate cancer is the second most common cancer in men worldwide. The older the man's age, the higher the risk of prostate cancer. About 80% of prostate cancer patients are men aged 65 and older. The incidence and mortality rate of prostate cancer is higher in Western countries compared to that in Asian countries. However, Asian immigrants to the United States, including Chinese and Japanese, increased the incidence rate of prostate cancer compared to that of their respective compatriots, which implies that Western diets may play a significant role in the incidence of prostate cancer.

What types of antioxidant foods can prevent prostate cancer?

Frequent consumption of tomato, soy foods, legumes, and cruciferous vegetables reduced the risk of prostate cancer. Table 55.1 illustrates that tomato consumption reduced the risk of prostate cancer by 14%. In addition, raw tomato reduced the risk of prostate cancer by 11%, and cooked tomato reduced the risk of prostate cancer by 19%. Moreover, the consumption of legumes and garlic reduced the risk of prostate cancer by 15% and 23%, respectively. Lastly, the consumption of tofu and cruciferous vegetables reduced the risk of prostate cancer by 30% and 22%, respectively.

Table 55.1.   Meta-analytical Confirmation of Antioxidant Food Remedies for Prostate Cancer

Antioxidant Foods	Reduced Risk, Prostate Cancer
Cruciferous vegetables	Cruciferous vegetables reduced the risk of prostate cancer by 22%.
Garlic	Garlic reduced the risk of prostate cancer by 23%.
Legumes	Legumes reduced the risk of prostate cancer by 15%. Each additional intake of 20 g of legumes per day reduced the risk by 3.5%.
Soy foods	Men who regularly consumed unfermented soy foods such as tofu reduced the risk of prostate cancer by 30%.
Tomatoes	Tomatoes reduced the risk of prostate cancer by 14%. Raw tomatoes and cooked tomatoes reduced the risk of prostate cancer by 11% and 19%, respectively.

56

Stomach Cancer

Globally, stomach cancer ranks the fourth most common cancer. According to the World Health Organization data, 770,000 people died from stomach cancer worldwide each year, and more than 50% of stomach cancer occurred in Asia regions, including Japan, China, Korea, Taiwan, and South Asia countries. In addition, about 10,000 people suffer from stomach cancer in the United States each year, and men are twice more likely than women to suffer from the disease.

What types of antioxidant foods can prevent stomach cancer?

Regular consumption of allium vegetables, dietary fiber, fruits, vegetables, and soy foods reduced the risk of stomach cancer, as shown in Table 56.1. Consumption of allium vegetables, such as garlic and onions, reduced the risk of stomach cancer by 46%. Further analysis showed that garlic consumption reduced the risk of stomach cancer by 40%, and onion consumption reduced the risk of stomach cancer by 45%. In addition, a daily intake of 10 g of dietary fiber reduced the risk of stomach cancer by 44%. Moreover, fruits and vegetables reduced the risk of stomach cancer in men and women by 11% and 17%, respectively, and a daily intake of 100 g of citrus fruits reduced the risk of stomach cancer by 40%. Furthermore, the consumption of cruciferous vegetables and carrots reduced the risk of stomach cancer by 19% and 26%, respectively. Finally, soy consumption reduced the risk of stomach cancer by 15–36%.

Table 56.1. Meta-analytical Confirmation of Antioxidant Food Remedies for Stomach Cancer

Antioxidant Foods	Reduced Risk, Stomach Cancer
Allium vegetables	Allium vegetables reduced the risk of stomach cancer by 46%. Among allium vegetables, garlic and onions reduced the risk of stomach cancer by 40% and 45%, respectively.
Citrus fruits	Each additional intake of 100 g of citrus fruits per day reduced the risk of stomach cancer by 40%.
Dietary fiber	Foods rich in dietary fiber reduced the risk of stomach cancer by 42%. Each additional dietary fiber intake of 10 g per day reduced the risk of stomach cancer by 44%.
Fruits and vegetables	Fruits and vegetables reduced the risk of stomach cancer in men and women by 11% and 17%, respectively.
Soy foods	Soy foods reduced the risk of stomach cancer by 15–36%.

What types of harmful foods can cause stomach cancer?

Habitual consumption of high-salt foods, pickled vegetables, red meat, and processed meat significantly elevated the risk of stomach cancer as shown in Table 56.2. Consumption of high-salt foods increased the risk of stomach cancer by 105%. Each additional intake of 1 teaspoon of salt per day increased the risk of stomach cancer by 12%. Pickled vegetables are a common staple food in many Asian countries, including Korea, China, and Japan. Consequently, Koreans, Chinese and Japanese who consumed pickled vegetables increased the risk of stomach cancer by 89%, 86%, and 16%, respectively. Furthermore, habitual consumption of red meat and processed meat increased the risk of stomach cancer by 67% and 76%, respectively. When analyzed one by one, beef and bacon increased the risk of stomach cancer by 28% and 37%, and ham and sausages increased the risk of stomach cancer by 44% and 33%, respectively.

Table 56.2. Meta-analytical Confirmation of Stomach Cancer-causative Foods

Harmful Foods	Increased Risk, Stomach Cancer
High salt	High-salt foods increased the risk of stomach cancer by 105%.
	Each additional intake of 5 g of salt per day increased the risk of stomach cancer by 12%.
Pickled vegetables	Pickled vegetables increased the risk of stomach cancer by 28%.
Processed meat	Processed meat increased the risk by 76%
Red meat	Red meat increased the risk by 67%.

57

Stroke

Stroke occurs when poor blood flow to the brain results in the death of neurons. Two types of stroke are ischemic stroke in which blood flowing to the brain is occluded by blood clots and hemorrhagic stroke in which blood flowing to the brain is interrupted due to bleeding. Every year, about 800,000 people suffer from stroke in the United States, of which 85% are ischemic stroke and the rest are hemorrhagic stroke. Stroke is the leading cause of vascular dementia and chronic disability. The major risk factors for stroke include hypertension, obesity, smoking, type 2 diabetes, heart disease, and hypercholesterolemia.

What types of antioxidant foods can prevent stroke?

Eight food items, including soy foods, olive oil, fruits, vegetables, whole grains, nuts, dietary fiber, fish, and dairy foods were effective in lowering the risk of stroke (see Table 57.1). Soy foods, olive oil, and whole grains reduced the risk of stroke by 46%, 17%, and 14%, respectively. Foods rich in dietary fiber reduced the risk of stroke by 13%. In addition, a high intake of dietary fiber reduced the risk of stroke by 20% in women and the risk of stroke by 5% in men. Consumption of fruits and vegetables reduced the risk of stroke by 21%. When analyzed separately, consumption of fruits reduced the risk of stroke by 32% and consumption of vegetables reduced the risk of stroke by 11%. Moreover, a daily intake of nuts reduced the risk of stroke by 16% in women and the risk of stroke by 12% in men. Habitual consumption of milk and cheese reduced the risk of

Table 57.1. Meta-analytical Confirmation of Antioxidant Food Remedies for Stroke

Antioxidant Foods	Reduced Risk, Stroke
Dietary fiber	Foods rich in dietary fiber reduced the risk of stroke by 13%. Each additional intake of 10 g of dietary fiber per day reduced the risk of stroke by 12%.
Fish	Fish intake of once per month, once per week, 2–4 times per week, and more than 5 times per week reduced the risk of stroke by 3%, 14%, 9%, and 13%, respectively.
Fruits	200 g of fruits daily reduced the risk of stroke by 32%.
Fruits and vegetables	Fruits and vegetables reduced the risk by 21%. Daily intake of 3 servings and 3–5 servings of fruits and vegetables reduced the risk of stroke by 11% and 26%, respectively.
Low-fat milk	200 ml of low-fat milk daily reduced the risk of stroke by 18%.
Nuts	Nuts reduced the risk of stroke in men and women by 12% and 16%, respectively. 12 g of mixed nuts daily reduced the risk of stroke by 14%.
Olive oil	Olive oil reduced the risk of stroke by 17%. 25 g of olive oil daily reduced the risk of stroke by 26%.
Soy foods	Soy foods reduced the risk of stroke by 46%.
Vegetables	200 g of vegetables daily reduced the risk of stroke by 11%.
Whole grains	Whole grains reduced the risk of stroke in men and women by 14% and 22%, respectively. 90 g of whole grains daily reduced the risk of stroke by 12%.

stroke by 18% and 5%, respectively. Lastly, the optimal amount of milk intake to provide the best protection against the incidence of stroke is 200 to 300 ml per day.

What types of harmful foods are linked to stroke?

High consumption of red meat, processed meat, high-salt foods, and artificially sweetened beverages exacerbated the incidence of stroke (see Table 57.2). Consumption of red meat and processed meat increased the risk of total stroke, cerebral infarction, and ischemic stroke by 14%, 13%, and 22%, respectively. When analyzed

Table 57.2.   Meta-analytical Confirmation of Stroke-causative Foods

Harmful Foods	Increased Risk, Stroke
Artificially sweetened beverages	Artificially-sweetened beverages increased the risk of total stroke and ischemic stroke by 14% and 19%, respectively.
High salt	High-salt foods increased the risk of stroke by 34%.
Processed meat	Processed meat increased the risk of total stroke and ischemic stroke by 14%–17% and 19%, respectively. Each additional intake of 50 g of processed meat increased the risk of stroke by 12%.
Red meat	Red meat increased the risk of total stroke and ischemic stroke by 9–13% and 13%, respectively. Each additional intake of 100 g of red meat increased the risk of stroke by 13%.
Red meat and processed meat	Red meat and processed meat increased the risk of total stroke, cerebral infarction stroke, and ischemic stroke by 14%, 13%, and 22%, respectively.

separately, red meat increased the risk of total stroke by 9–13% and the risk of ischemic stroke by 13%, while processed meat increased the risk of total stroke by 14–17% and the risk of ischemic stroke by 19%. Quantitative studies showed that a daily consumption of a piece of 4 ounces of steak increased the risk of stroke by 13%, and a daily consumption of 2 pieces of bacon increased the risk of stroke by 11%. In addition, habitual consumption of high-salt foods increased the risk of stroke by 34%. Lastly, high consumption of artificially sweetened beverages increased the risk of total stroke by 14% and the risk of ischemic stroke by 19%.

58

Type 2 Diabetes

Type 2 diabetes is a chronic disease characterized by the body's inability to metabolize glucose. In a healthy person, glucose is metabolized in the cells to produce energy, and in a diabetic patient, glucose cannot be efficiently metabolized, and result in insufficient energy production. The symptoms of type 2 diabetes include frequent urination, thirst, hungry, fatigue, blurred vision, and weight loss. Globally, about 6.4% of all adults are inflicted with type 2 diabetes. It is estimated that by the year 2030, more than 400 million people worldwide will suffer from type 2 diabetes. Type 2 diabetes is a leading cause of heart disease and stroke, and its complications include chronic kidney disease and blindness.

What types of antioxidant foods may alleviate type 2 diabetes?

The meta-analytical results have identified ten anti-diabetic food items, including aloe vera, whole grains, cinnamon, garlic, probiotics, dietary fiber, fruits, vegetables, low-fat milk, and nuts (see Table 58.1). Consumption of aloe vera reduced the fasting glucose level by 21.1 mg/dL and HbA1c by 1.1% in type 2 diabetic patients. Aloe vera intake also reduced the fasting glucose level by 4 mg/dL in pre-diabetic individuals. Consumption of three servings of whole grains (15 g per serving) daily reduced the risk of type 2 diabetes by 20% in pre-diabetic individuals, and the consumption of cinnamon decreased the fasting glucose level by 24.6 mg/dL in type 2 diabetic patients. In addition, the consumption of garlic decreased the fasting glucose level by 17.3 mg/dL in type 2 diabetic patients and decreased fasting glucose by 2 mg/dL in pre-diabetic individuals.

Table 58.1. Meta-analytical Confirmation of Antioxidant Food Remedies for Type 2 Diabetes

Antioxidant Foods	Treat/Reduce Risk, Type 2 Diabetes
Aloe vera	Aloe vera decreased fasting glucose level by 21.1 mg/dL and HbA1c by 1.1 % in type 2 diabetic patients. Aloe vera decreased fasting glucose level by 4 mg/dL in pre-diabetic individuals.
Cheese	50 g of cheese daily reduced the risk of type 2 diabetes by 8%.
Cinnamon	120 mg of cinnamon powder daily for 4–18 weeks reduced fasting glucose level by 24.6 mg/dL in type 2 diabetic patients. 1–6 g of cinnamon daily for 40 days to 4 months reduced fasting glucose level by 15.3 mg/dL and HbA1C by 0.09% in type 2 diabetic patients.
Dietary fiber	Dietary fiber reduced fasting glucose level by 9.97 mg/dL and HbA1c by 0.55% in type 2 diabetic patients. Whole grain dietary fiber, fruit dietary fiber, and vegetable dietary fiber reduced the risk of type 2 diabetes in pre-diabetic individuals by 25%, 5%, and 7%, respectively.
Fruits	Fruits reduced the risk of type 2 diabetes by 7%. Among fruits, blueberries and apples/pears reduced the risk of type 2 diabetes by 25% and 18%, respectively. 200 g of fruits daily reduced the risk of type 2 diabetes by 13%.
Garlic	Garlic reduced fasting glucose level by 17.3 mg/dL in type 2 diabetic patients. Garlic reduced fasting glucose level by 1.7 mg/dL in pre-diabetic individuals.
Low-fat milk	Daily intake of 200 ml of low-fat milk reduced the risk of type 2 diabetes by 9%.
Nuts	Diabetic patients who consumed 56 g of mixed nuts per day reduced fasting glucose level by 2.7 mg/dL. Pre-diabetic individuals who consumed 28.4 g of mixed nuts per day reduced the risk by13%.
Olive oil	Olive oil reduced fasting glucose level by 8 mg/dL and HbA1c 0.3% in type 2 diabetic patients. Olive oil reduced the risk of type 2 diabetes by16% in pre-diabetic individuals.

(Continued)

Table 58.1.   (*Continued*)

Antioxidant Foods	Treat/Reduce Risk, Type 2 Diabetes
Probiotics	Probiotics reduced fasting glucose level by 9.5 mg/dL and HbA1c by 0.32% in type 2 diabetic patients.
Vegetables	Vegetables reduced the risk of type 2 diabetes by 10%. Separately, dark green leafy vegetables, white vegetables, and cruciferous vegetables reduced the risk of type 2 diabetes by 23%, 38%, and 38%, respectively.
Whole grains	3 servings of whole grains (15 g per serving) daily reduced the risk of type 2 diabetes by 20%.
Yogurt	80 g of yogurt daily reduced the risk of type 2 diabetes by 14%.

Moreover, probiotics decreased the fasting glucose level by 9.5 mg/dL and HbA1c by 0.32% in type 2 diabetic patients and dietary fiber decreased the fasting glucose level by 9.97 mg/dL and HbA1c by 0.55% in type 2 diabetic patients. When analyzed separately, consumption of whole grain dietary fiber, fruit dietary fiber, and vegetable dietary fiber reduced the risk of incident type 2 diabetes by 25%, 5% and 7%, respectively. Among all dietary fibers, whole grain fiber appears to be most effective in lowering the risk of type 2 diabetes.

Intake of olive oil decreased the fasting glucose level by 8 mg/dL and HbA1c by 0.3% in type 2 diabetic patients. Consumption of fruits and vegetables reduced the risk of type 2 diabetes by 7%. Among different vegetables, dark green leafy vegetables, white vegetables, and cruciferous vegetables reduced the risk of type 2 diabetes by 23%, 38% and 38%, respectively. Among different fruits, blueberries and apples/pears reduced the risk of type 2 diabetes by 25% and 18%. Lastly, a daily consumption of low-fat milk, yogurt, and whole milk reduced the risk of type 2 diabetes by 9%, 14%, and 8%, respectively.

What types of harmful foods can cause type 2 diabetes?

Habitual consumption of white rice, red meat, processed meat, egg, sugar-sweetened beverages, artificially-sweetened beverages,

Table 58.2.   Meta-analytical Confirmation of Type 2 Diabetes-causative Foods

Harmful Foods	Increased Risk, Type 2 Diabetes
Artificially-sweetened beverage	Each additional serving of artificially-sweetened beverages per day increased the risk of type 2 diabetes by 8%.
Eggs	2 or more eggs per week increased the risk of type 2 diabetes by 18%.
	4 or more eggs per week increased the risk of type 2 diabetes by 29%.
Fruit juice	Each additional serving of sugar-sweetened fruit juice per day increased the risk of type 2 diabetes by 7%.
Processed meat	Processed meat increased the risk of type 2 diabetes by 51%.
	Each additional intake of 50 g of processed meat per day increased the risk of type 2 diabetes by 19%.
Red meat	Red meat increased the risk of type 2 diabetes by 14%.
	100 g of red meat daily increased fasting glucose level by 0.67 mg/dL.
	Each additional intake of 100 g of red meat per day increased the risk of type 2 diabetes by 19%.
Sugar-sweetened beverage	Each additional intake of 1–2 cans of sugar-sweetened beverages per day increased the risk of type 2 diabetes by 26%.
White rice	White rice increased the risk of type 2 diabetes in Asian people and Western people by 55% and 12%, respectively.
	Each additional serving of white rice per day increased the risk of type 2 diabetes by 11%.

and sugar-sweetened fruit juice greatly increased the risk of type 2 diabetes (see Table 58.2). High consumption of white rice increased the risk of type 2 diabetes by 55%. Processed meat raised risk of type 2 diabetes by 51%, while red meat heightened the risk of type 2 diabetes by 14%. In addition, consumption of 4 or more eggs per week increased the risk of type 2 diabetes by 29%. Moreover, high consumption of sugar-sweetened beverages, artificially-sweetened beverages, and fruit juice increased the risk of type 2 diabetes by 13%, 8% and 7%, respectively.

Author's Publications

Komarov A, Mattson D, Jones MM, Singh PK, Lai CS. (1993) *In vivo* spin trapping of nitric oxide in mice. *Biochem Biophys Res Commun* **195**:1191–1198.

Komarov AM, Lai CS. (1995) Detection of nitric oxide production in mice by spin-trapping electron paramagnetic resonance spectroscopy. *Biochim Biophys Acta* **1272**(1):29–36.

Lai CS, Komarov AM. (1994) Spin trapping of nitric oxide produced *in vivo* in septic shock mice. *FEBS Letters* **345**(2–3):120–124.

References

Breast cancer

Anderson JJ, Darwis NDM, Mackay DF, Celis-Morales CA, Lyall DM, Sattar N, Gill JMR, Pell JP. (2018) Red and processed meat consumption and breast cancer: UK Biobank cohort study and meta-analysis. *Eur J Cancer* **90**:73–82.

Aune D, Chan DS, Greenwood DC, Vieira AR, Rosenblatt DA, Vieira R, Norat T. (2012) Dietary fiber and breast cancer risk: a systematic review and meta-analysis of prospective studies. *Ann Oncol* **23**(6):1394–402.

Chen M, Rao Y, Zheng Y, Wei S, Li Y, Guo T, Yin P. (2014) Association between soy isoflavone intake and breast cancer risk for pre- and post-menopausal women: a meta-analysis of epidemiological studies. *PLoS One* **9**(2):e89288.

Chen S, Chen Y, Ma S, Zheng R, Zhao P, Zhang L, Liu Y, Yu Q, Deng Q, Zhang K. (2016) Dietary fibre intake and risk of breast cancer: a systematic review and meta-analysis of epidemiological studies. *Oncotarget* **7**(49):80980–9.

Chi F, Wu R, Zeng YC, Xing R, Liu Y, Xu ZG. (2013) Post-diagnosis soy food intake and breast cancer survival: a meta-analysis of cohort studies. *Asian Pac J Cancer Prev* **14**(4):2407–12.

Dong JY, He K, Wang P, Qin LQ. (2011) Dietary fiber intake and risk of breast cancer: a meta-analysis of prospective cohort studies. *Am J Clin Nutr* **94**(3):900–5.

Dong JY, Qin LQ. (2011) Soy isoflavones consumption and risk of breast cancer incidence or recurrence: a meta-analysis of prospective studies. *Breast Cancer Res Treat* **125**(2):315–23.

Dong JY, Zhang L, He K, Qin LQ. (2011) Dairy consumption and risk of breast cancer: a meta-analysis of prospective cohort studies. *Breast Cancer Res Treat* **127**(1):23–31.

Fabiani R, Minelli L, Rosignoli P. (2016) Apple intake and cancer risk: a systematic review and meta-analysis of observational studies. *Public Health Nutr* **19**(14):2603–17.

He J, Gu Y, Zhang S. (2017) Consumption of vegetables and fruits and breast cancer survival: a systematic review and meta-analysis. *Sci Rep* **7**(1):599.

Hui C, Qi X, Qianyong Z, Xiaoli P, Jundong Z, Mantian M. (2013) Flavonoids, flavonoid subclasses and breast cancer risk: the meta-analysis of epidemiological studies. *PLoS One* **8**(1):e54318.

Keum N, Lee DH, Marchand N, Oh H, Liu H, Aune D, Greenwood DC, Giovannucci EL. (2015) Egg intake and cancers of the breast, ovary and prostate: a dose-response meta-analysis of prospective observational studies. *Br J Nutr* **114**(7):1099–107.

Liu X, Lv K. (2013) Cruciferous vegetables intake is inversely associated with risk of breast cancer: a meta-analysis. *Breast* **22**(3):309–13.

Liu XO, Huang YB, Gao Y, Chen C, Yan Y, Dai HJ, Song FJ, Wang YG, Wang PS, Chen KX. (2014) Association between dietary factors and breast cancer risk among Chinese females: systematic review and meta-analysis. *Asian Pac J Cancer Prev* **15**(3):1291–8.

Nindrea RD, Aryandono T, Lazuardi L, Dwiprahasto I. (2019) Protective effect of omega-3 fatty acids in fish consumption against breast cancer in Asian patients: A meta-analysis. *Asian Pac J Cancer Prev* **20**:327–32.

Schwingshackl L, Hoffmann G. (2015) Adherence to Mediterranean diet and risk of cancer: an updated systematic review and meta-analysis of observational studies. *Cancer Med* **4**(12):1933–47.

Si R, Qu K, Jiang Z, Yang X, Gao P. (2014) Egg consumption and breast cancer risk: the meta-analysis. *Breast Cancer* **21**(3):251–61.

Song K, Bae JM. (2013) Citrus fruit intake and breast cancer risk: a quantitative systematic review. *J Breast Cancer* **16**(1):72–6.

Van den Brandt PA, Schulpen M. (2017) Mediterranean diet adherence and risk of postmenopausal breast cancer: results of a cohort study and meta-analysis. *Int J Cancer* **140**(10):2220–31.

Wu J, Zeng R, Huang J, Li X, Zhang J, Ho JC, Zheng Y. (2016) Dietary protein sources and incidence of breast cancer: a dose-response meta-analysis of prospective studies. *Nutrients* **8**(11):pii: E730.

Wu YC, Zheng D, Sun JJ, Zou ZK, Ma ZL. (2015) Meta-analysis of studies on breast cancer risk and diet in Chinese women. *Int J Clin Exp Med* **8**(1):73–85.

Zang J, Shen M, Du S, Chen T, Zou S. (2015) The association between dairy intake and breast cancer in Western and Asian populations: a systematic review and meta-analysis. *J Breast Cancer* **18**(4):313–22.

Zhao TT, Jin F, Li JG, Xu YY, Dong HT, Liu Q, Xing P, Zhu GL, Xu H, Miao ZF. (2019) Dietary isoflavones or isoflavone-rich food intake and breast cancer risk: a meta-analysis of prospective studies. *Clin Nutr* **38**(1):136–45.

Cardiovascular disease

Alexander DD, Bylsma LC, Vargas AJ, Cohen SS, Doucette A, Mohamed M, Irvin SR, Miller PE, Watson H, Fryzek JP. (2006) Dairy consumption and CVD: a systematic review and meta-analysis. *Br J Nutr* **115**(4): 737–50.

Aune D, Keum N, Giovannucci E, Fadnes LT, Boffetta P, Greenwood DC, Tonstad S, Vatten LJ, Riboli E, Norat T. (2016) Whole grain consumption and risk of cardiovascular disease, and all cause and cause specific mortality: systematic review and dose-response meta-analysis of prospective studies. *BMJ* **353**:i2716.

Aune D. Giovannucci E, Boffetta P, Fadnes LT, Keum N, Norat T, Greenwood DC, Riboli E, Vatten LJ, Tonstad S. (2017) Fruit and vegetable intake and the risk of cardiovascular disease, total cancer and all-cause mortality-a systematic review and dose-re-sponse meta-analysis of prospective studies. *Int J Epidermol* **46**(3):1029–56.

Beavers DP, Beavers KM, Miller M, Stamey J, Messina MJ. (2012) Exposure to isoflavone-containing soy products and endothelial function: a Bayesian meta-analysis of randomized controlled trials. *Nutr Metab Cardiovasc Dis* **22**(3):182–91.

Cheng HM, Koutsidis G, Lodge JK, Ashor A, Siervo M, Lara J. (2017) Tomato and lycopene supplementation and cardiovascular risk factors: a systematic review and meta-analysis. *Atherosclerosis* **257**:100–8.

Cheng HM, Koutsidis G, Lodge JK, Ashor AW, Siervo M, Lara J. (2019) Lycopene and tomato and risk of cardiovascular diseases: a systematic review and meta-analysis. *Crit Rev Food Sci Nutr* **59**(1):141–58.

Chowdhury R, Stevens S, Gorman D, Pan A, Warnakula S, Chowdhury S, Ward H, Johnson L, Crowe F, Hu FB, Franco OH. (2012) Association between fish consumption, long chain omega 3 fatty acids, and risk of cerebrovascular disease: systematic review and meta-analysis. *BMJ* **345**:e6698.

Daroohegi Mofrad M, Milajerdi A, Koh Dani F, Surkan PJ, Azadbakt L. (2019) Garlic supplementation reduces circulating C-reactive protein, tumor necrosis factor and interleukin-6 in adults: a systematic review and meta-analysis of randomized controlled trials. *J Nutr* **149**(4):605–18.

Feringa HH, Laskey DA, Dickson JE, Coleman CI. (2011) The effect of grape seed extract on cardiovascular risk markers: a meta-analysis of randomized controlled trials. *J Am Diet Assoc* **111**(8):1173–81.

Grosso G, Marventano S, Yang J, Micek A, Pajak A, Scalfi L, Galvano F, Kales SN. (2017) A comprehensive meta-analysis of Mediterranean diet and cardiovascular disease: Are individual components equal? *Crit Rev Food Sci Nutr* **57**(15):3218–32.

Hohmann CD, Cramer H, Michalsen A, Kessler C, Steckhan N, Choi K, Dobos G. (2015) Effects of high phenolic olive oil on cardiovascular risk factors: a systematic review and meta-analysis. *Phytomedicine* **22**(6):631–40.

Huang H, Chen G, Liao D, Zhu Y, Xue X. (2016) Effects of berries consumption on cardiovascular risk factors: a meta-analysis with trial sequential analysis of randomized controlled trials. *Sci Rep* **6**:23625.

Jayedi A, Zargar MS, Shab-Bidar S. (2019) Fish consumption and risk of myocarfdial infarction: a systematic review and dose-response meta-analysis suggests a regional difference. *Nutr Res* **62**:1–12.

Kwak JS, Kim JY, Paek JE, Lee YJ, Kim HR, Park DS, Kwon O. (2014) Garlic powder intake and cardiovascular risk factors: a meta-analysis of randomized controlled clinical trials. *Nutr Res Pract* 8(6):644–54.

Li SH, Tian HB, Zhao HJ, Chen LH, Cui LQ. (2013) The acute effects of grape polyphenols supplementation on endothelial function in adults: meta-analysis of controlled trials. *PLoS One* 8(7):e69818.

Liyanage T, Ninomiya T, Wang A, Neal B, Jun M, Wong MG, Jardine M, Hillis GS, Perkovic V. (2016) Effects of the Mediterranean diet on cardiovascular outcomes: a systematic review and meta-analysis. *PLoS One* 11(8):e0159252.

Mayhew AJ, de Souza RJ, Meyre D, Anand SS, Mente A. (2016) A systematic review and meta-analysis of nut consumption and incident risk of CVD and all-cause mortality. *Br J Nutr* 115(2):212–25.

Marventano S, Izquierdo Pulido M, Sanchez-Gonzalez C, Godos J, Speciani A, Galvano F, Grosso G. (2017) Legume consumption and CVD risk: a systematic review and meta-analysis. *Public Health Nutr* 20(2):245–54.

McRae MP. (2017) Health benefits of dietary whole grains: an umbrella review of meta-analysis. *J Chiropr Med* 16(1):10–8.

Narain A, Kwok CS, Mamas MA. (2016) Soft drinks and sweetened beverages and the risk of cardiovascular disease and mortality: a systematic review and meta-analysis. *Int J Clin Pract* 70(10):791–805.

Pollock RL. (2016) The effect of green leafy and cruciferous vegetable intake on the incidence of cardiovascular disease: a meta-analysis. *JRSM Cardiovasc Dis* 5:2048004016661435.

Qin LQ, Xu JY, Han SF, Zhang ZL, Zhao YY, Szeto IM. (2015) Dairy consumption and risk of cardiovascular disease: an updated meta-analysis of prospective cohort studies. *Asia Pac J Clin Nutr* 24(1):90–100.

Schwingshackl L, Hoffmann G. (2014) Monounsaturated fatty acids, olive oil and health status: a systematic review and meta-analysis of cohort studies: *Lipids Health Dis* 13:154.

Schwingshackl L, Christoph M, Hoffmann G. (2015) Effects of olive oil on markers of inflammation and endothelial function — a systematic review and meta-analysis. *Nutrients* 7(9):7651–75.

Strazzullo P, D'Elia L, Kandala NB, Cappuccio FP. (2009) Salt intake, stroke, and cardiovascular disease: meta-analysis of prospective studies. *BMJ* **339**:b4567.

Threapleton DE, Greenwood DC, Evans CE, Cleghorn CL, Nykjaer C, Woodhead C, Cade JE, Gale CP, Burley VJ. (2013) Dietary fibre intake and risk of cardiovascular disease: systematic review and meta-analysis. *BMJ* **347**:f6879.

Veronese N, Solmi M, Caruso MG, Giannelli G, Osella AR, Evangelou E, Maggi S, Fontana L, Stubbs B, Tzoulaki I. (2018) Dietary fiber and health outcomes: an umbrella review of systematic reviews and meta-analyses. *Am J Clin Nutr* **107**(3):436–44.

Yan Z, Zhang X, Li C, Jiao S, Dong W. (2017) Association between consumption of soy and risk of cardiovascular disease: a meta-analysis of observational studies. *Eur J Prev Cardiol* **24**(7):735–47.

Ye EQ, Chacko SA, Chou EL, Kugizaki M, Liu S. (2012) Greater whole-grain intake is associated with lower risk of type 2 diabetes, cardiovascular disease, and weight gain. *J Nutr* **142**(7):1304–13.

Zhan J, Liu YJ, Cai LB, Xu FR, Xie T, He QQ. (2017) Fruit and vegetable consumption and risk of cardiovascular disease: a meta-analysis of prospective cohort studies. *Crit Rev Food Sci Nutr* **57**(8):1650–63.

Chronic kidney disease

Cheungpasitporn W, Thongprayoon C, O'Corragain OA, Edmonds PJ, Kittanamongkochai W, Erickson SB. (2014) Associations of sugar-sweetened and artificially sweetened soda with chronic kidney disease: a systematic review and meta-analysis. *Nephrology (Carlton)* **19**(12):791–7.

Chiavaroli L, Mirrahimi A, Sievenpiper JL, Jenkins DJ, Darling PB. (2015) Dietary fiber effects in chronic kidney disease: a systematic review and meta-analysis of controlled feeding trials. *Eur J Clin Nutr* **69**(7):761–8.

Jing Z, Wei-Jie Y. (2016) Effects of soy protein containing isoflavones in patients with chronic kidney disease: a systematic review and meta-analysis. *Clin Nutr* **35**(1):117–24.

Kovesdy CP, Kalantar-Zadeh K. (2016) Back to the future: restricted protein intake for conservative management of CKD, triple goals of renoprotection, uremia mitigation and nutritional health. *Int Urol Nephrol* **48**(5):725–9.

Liu N, Sun W, Xing Z, Ma F, Sun T, Wu H, Dong Y, Xu Z, Fu Y, Yuan H. (2015) Association between sodium intakes with the risk of chronic kidney disease: evidence from the meta-analysis. *Int J Clin Exp Med* **8**(11):20939–45.

Oyabu C, Hashimoto Y, Fukuda T, Tanaka M, Asano M, Yamazaki M, Fukui M. (2016) Impact of low-carbohydrate diet on renal function: the meta-analysis of over 1000 individuals from nine randomized controlled trials. *Br J Nutr* **116**(4):632–8.

Rhee CM, Ahmadi SF, Kovesdy CP, Kalantar-Zadeh K. (2018) Low-protein diet for conservative management of chronic kidney disease: a systematic review and meta-analysis of controlled trials. *J Cachexia Sarcopenia Muscle* **9**(2):235–45.

Rughooputh MS, Zeng R, Yao Y. (2015) Protein diet restriction slows chronic kidney disease progression in non-diabetic and in type 1 diabetic patients, but not in type 2 diabetic patients: a meta-analysis of randomized controlled trials using glomerular filtration rate as a surrogate. *PLoS One* **10**(12):e0145505.

Zhang J, Liu J, Su J, Tian F. (2014) The effects of soy protein on chronic kidney disease: a meta-analysis of randomized controlled trials. *Eur J Clin Nutr* **68**(9):987–93.

Cognitive impairment

Bakre AT, Chen R, Khutan R, Wei L, Smith T, Qin G, Danat IM, Zhou W, Schofield P, Clifford A, Wang J, Verma A, Zhang C, Ni J. (2018) Association between fish consumption and risk of dementia: a new study from China and a systematic literature review and meta-analysis. *Public Health Nutr* **21**(10):1921–32.

Cao L, Tan L, Wang HF, Jiang T, Zhu XC, Lu H, Tan MS, Yu JT. (2016) Dietary patterns and risk of dementia: a systematic review and meta-analysis of cohort studies. *Mol Neurobiol* **53**(9):6144–54.

Cheng PF, Chen JJ, Zhou XY, Ren YF, Huang W, Zhou JJ, Xie P. (2015) Do soy isoflavones improve cognitive function in postmenopausal women? A meta-analysis. *Menopause* **22**(2):198–206.

Jiang X, Huang J, Song D, Deng R, Wei J, Zhang Z. (2017) Increased consumption of fruit and vegetables is related to a reduced risk of cognitive impairment and dementia: meta-analysis. *Front Aging Neurosci* **9**:18.

Radd-Vagenas S, Duffy SL, Naismith SL, Brew BJ, Flood VM, Fiatarone Singh MA. (2018) Effect of the Mediterranean diet on cognition and brain morphology and function: a systematic review of randomized controlled trials. *Am J Clin Nutr* **107**(3):389–404.

Wu L, Sun D. (2016) Meta-analysis of milk consumption and the risk of cognitive disorders: *Nutrients* **8**(12):pii: E824.

Wu L, Sun D. (2017) Adherence to Mediterranean diet and risk of developing cognitive disorders: an updated systematic review and meta-analysis of prospective cohort studies. *Sci Rep* **7**:41317.

Xu W, Wang H, Wan Y, Tan C, Li J, Tan L, Yu JT. (2017) Alcohol consumption and dementia risk: a dose-response meta-analysis of prospective studies. *Eur J Epidemiol* **32**(1):31–42.

Zeng LF, Cao Y, Liang WX, Bao WH, Pan JK, Wang Q, Liu J, Liang HD, Xie H, Chai YT, Guan ZT, Cao Q, Li XY, Yang L, Xu WH, Mi SQ, Wang NS. (2017) An exploration of the role of a fish-oriented diet in cognitive decline: a systematic review of the literature. *Oncotarget* **8**(24):39877–95.

Zhang Y, Chen J, Qiu J, Li Y, Wang J, Jiao J. (2016) Intakes of fish and polyunsaturated fatty acids and mild-to-severe cognitive impairment risks: a dose-response meta-analysis of 21 cohort studies. *Am J Clin Nutr* **103**(2):330–40.

Colorectal cancer

Aune D, Chan DS, Lau R, Vieira R, Greenwood DC, Kampman E, Norat T. (2011) Dietary fibre, whole grains, and risk of colorectal cancer: systematic review and dose-response meta-analysis of prospective studies. *BMJ* **343**:d6617.

Aune D, Chan DS, Vieira AR, Navarro Rosenblatt DA, Vieira R, Greenwood DC, Kampman E, Norat T. (2013) Red and processed meat intake and risk of colorectal adenomas: a systematic review and meta-analysis of epidemiological studies. *Cancer Causes Control* **24**(4):611–27.

Aune D, Lau R, Chan DS, Vieira R, Greenwood DC, Kampman E, Norat T. (2012) Dairy products and colorectal cancer risk: a systematic review and meta-analysis of cohort studies. *Ann Oncol* **23**(1):37–45.

Ben Q, Sun Y, Chai R, Qian A, Xu B, Yuan Y. (2014) Dietary fiber intake reduces risk for colorectal adenoma: a meta-analysis. *Gastroenterology* **146**(3):689–99.

Ben Q, Zhong J, Liu J, Wang L, Sun Y, Yv L, Yuan Y. (2015) Association between consumption of fruits and vegetables and risk of colorectal adenoma: a PRISMA-compliant meta-analysis of observational studies. *Medicine (Baltimore)* **94**(42):e1599.

Carr PR, Walter V, Brenner H, Hoffmeister M. (2016) Meat subtypes and their association with colorectal cancer: systematic review and meta-analysis. *Int J Cancer* **138**(2):293–302.

Cho E, Smith-Warner SA, Spiegelman D, Beeson WL, van den Brandt PA, Colditz GA, Folsom AR, Fraser GE, Freudenheim JL, Giovannucci E, Goldbohm RA, Graham S, Miller AB, Pietinen P, Potter JD, Rohan TE, Terry P, Toniolo P, Virtanen MJ, Willett WC, Wolk A, Wu K, Yaun SS, Zeleniuch-Jacquotte A, Hunter DJ. (2004) Dairy foods, calcium, and colorectal cancer: a pooled analysis of 10 cohort studies. *J Natl Cancer Inst* **96**(13):1015–22.

Feng YL, Shu L, Zheng PF, Zhang XY, Si CJ, Yu XL, Gao W, Zhang L. (2017) Dietary patterns and colorectal cancer risk: a meta-analysis. *Eur J Cancer Prev* **26**(3):201–11.

Geelen A, Schouten JM, Kamphuis C, Stam BE, Burema J, Renkema JM, Bakker EJ, van't Veer P, Kampman E. (2007) Fish consumption, n-3 fatty acids, and colorectal cancer: a meta-analysis of prospective cohort studies. *Am J Epidemiol* **166**(10):1116–25.

Gianfredi V, Salvatori T, Villarini M, Moretti M, Nucci D, Realdon S. (2018) Is dietary fibre truly protective against colon cancer? A systematic review and meta-analysis. *Int J Food Sci Nutr* **69**(8):904–15.

Godos J, Bella F, Torrisi A, Sciacca S, Galvano F, Grosso G. (2016) Dietary patterns and risk of colorectal adenoma: a systematic review and meta-analysis of observational studies. *J Hum Nutr Diet* **29**(6):757–67.

Haas P, Machado MJ, Anton AA, Silva AS, de Francisco A. (2009) Effectiveness of whole grain consumption in the prevention of colorectal cancer: meta-analysis of cohort studies. *Int J Food Sci Nutr* **60** Suppl 6:1–13.

Huncharek M, Muscat J, Kupelnick B. (2009) Colorectal cancer risk and dietary intake of calcium, vitamin D, and dairy products: a meta-analysis of 26,335 cases from 60 observational studies. *Nutr Cancer* **61**(1):47–69.

Jiang R, Botma A, Rudolph A, Husing A, Chang-Claude J. (2016) Phyto-oestrogens and colorectal cancer risk: a systematic review and dose-response meta-analysis of observational studies. *Br J Nutr* **116**(12):2115–28.

Johnson CM, Wei C, Ensor JE, Smolenski DJ, Amos CI, Levin B, Berry DA. (2016) Meta-analyses of colorectal cancer risk factors. *Cancer Causes Control* **24**(6):1207–22.

Lippi G, Mattiuzzi C, Cervellin G. (2016) Meat consumption and cancer risk: a critical review of published meta-analyses. *Crit Rev Oncol Hematol* **97**:1–14.

Magalhaes B, Peleteiro B, Lunet N. (2012) Dietary patterns and colorectal cancers: systematic review and meta-analysis. *Eur J Cancer Prev* **21**(1):15–23.

Ralston RA, Truby H, Palermo CE, Walker KZ. (2014) Colorectal cancer and nonfermented milk, solid cheese, and fermented milk consumption: a systematic review and meta-analysis of prospective studies. *Crit Rev Food Sci Nutr* **54**(9):1167–79.

Schwingshackl L, Schwedhelm C, Hoffmann G, Knuppel S, Laure Preterre A, Igbal K, Bechthold A, De Henauw S, Michels N, Devleesschauwer B, Boeing H, Schlesinger S. (2018) Food groups and risk of colorectal cancer. *Int J. Cancer* **142**(9):1748–58.

Tse G, Eslick GD. (2016) Soy and isoflavone consumption and risk of gastrointestinal cancer: a systematic review and meta-analysis. *Eur J Nutr* **55**(1):63–73.

Tse G, Eslick GD. (2014) Cruciferous vegetables and risk of colorectal neoplasms: a systematic review and meta-analysis. *Nutr Cancer* 66(1):128–39.

Tse G, Eslick GD. (2014) Egg consumption and risk of GI neoplasms: dose-response meta-analysis and systematic review. *Eur J Nutr* 53(7):1581–90.

Turati F, Guercio V, Pelucchi C, La Vecchia C, Galeone C. (2014) Colorectal cancer and adenomatous polyps in relation to allium vegetables intake: a meta-analysis of observational studies. *Mol Nutr Food Res* 58(9):1907–14.

Vieira AR, Abar L, Chan DSM, Vingeliene S, Polemiti E, Stevens C, Greenwood D, Norat T. (2017) Foods and beverages and colorectal cancer risk: a systematic review and meta-analysis of cohort studies, an update of the evidence of the WCRF-AICR continuous update project. *Ann Oncol* 28(8):1788–1802.

Wu S, Feng B, Li K, Zhu X, Liang S, Liu X, Han S, Wang B, Wu K, Miao D, Liang J, Fan D. (2012) Fish consumption and colorectal cancer risk in humans: a systematic review and meta-analysis. *Am J Med* 125(6):551–9.

Wu QJ, Yang Y, Vogtmann E, Wang J, Han LH, Li HL, Xiang YB. (2013) Cruciferous vegetables intake and the risk of colorectal cancer: a meta-analysis of observational studies. *Ann Oncol* 24(4):1079–87.

Xu X, Yu E, Gao X, Song N, Liu L, Wei X, Zhang W, Fu C. (2013) Red and processed meat intake and risk of colorectal adenomas: a meta-analysis of observational studies. *Int J Cancer* 132(2):437–48.

Yan L, Spitznagel EL, Bosland MC. (2010) Soy consumption and colorectal cancer risk in humans: a meta-analysis. *Cancer Epidemiol Biomarkers Prev* 19(1):148–58.

Yu Y, Jing X, Li H, Zhao X, Wang D. (2016) Soy isoflavone consumption and colorectal cancer risk: a systematic review and meta-analysis. *Sci Rep* 6:25939.

Yu XF, Zou J, Dong J. (2014) Fish consumption and risk of gastrointestinal cancers: a meta-analysis of cohort studies. *World J Gastroenterol* 20(41):15398–412.

Zhu B, Sun Y, Qi L, Zhong R, Miao X. (2015) Dietary legume consumption reduces risk of colorectal cancer: evidence from a meta-analysis of cohort studies. *Sci Rep* 5:8797.

Endometrial cancer

Bandera EV, Kushi LH, Moore DF, Gifkins DM, McCullough ML. (2007) Association between dietary fiber and endometrial cancer: a dose-response meta-analysis. *Am J Clin Nutr* **86**(6):1730–7.

Bandera EV, Kushi LH, Moore DF, Gifkins DM, McCullough ML. (2007) Fruits and vegetables and endometrial cancer risk: a systematic literature review and meta-analysis. *Nutr Cancer* **58**(1):6–21.

Gnagnarella P, Gandini S, La Vecchia C, Maisonneuve P. (2008) Glycemic index, glycemic load, and cancer risk: a meta-analysis. *Am J Clin Nutr* **87**(6):1793–801.

Jiang L, Hou R, Gong TT, Wu QJ. (2015) Dietary fat intake and endometrial cancer risk: dose-response meta-analysis of epidemiological studies. *Sci Rep* **5**:16693.

Mulholland HG, Murray LJ, Cardwell CR, Cantwell MM. (2008) Dietary glycaemic index, glycaemic load and endometrial and ovarian cancer risk: a systematic review and meta-analysis. *Br J Cancer* **99**(3):434–41.

Nagle CM, Olsen CM, Ibiebele TI, Spurdle AB, Webb PM. (2013) Australian National Endometrial Cancer Study Group; Australian Ovary Cancer Study Group. Glycemic index, glycemic load, and endometrial cancer risk; results from Australian National Endometrial Cancer Study and an updated systematic review and meta-analysis. *Eur J Nutr* **52**(2):705–15.

Zhang GQ, Chen JL, Liu Q, Zhang Y, Zeng H, Zhao Y. (2015) Soy intake is associated with lower endometrial cancer risk: a systematic review and meta-analysis of observational studies. *Medicine (Baltimore)* **94**(50):e2281.

Zhao J, Lyu C, Gao J, Du L, Shan B, Zhang H, Wang HY, Gao Y. (2016) Dietary fat intake and endometrial cancer risk: a dose-response meta-analysis. *Medicine (Baltimore)* **95**(27):e4121.

Zhong XS, Ge J, Chen SW, Xiong YQ, Ma SJ, Chen Q. (2018) Association between dietary isoflavones in soy and legumes and endometrial cancer: a systematic review and meta-analysis. *J Acad Nutr Diet* **118**(4):637–51.

Esophageal cancer

Akhtar S. (2013) Areca nut chewing and esophageal squamous-cell carcinoma risk in Asians: a meta-analysis case-control studies, *Cancer Causes Control* **24**(2):257–65.

Choi Y, Song S, Song Y, Lee JE. (2013) Consumption of red and processed meat and esophageal cancer risk: meta-analysis. *World J Gastroenterol* **19**(7):1020–9.

Coleman HG, Murray LJ, Hicks B, Bhat SK, Kubo A, Corley DA, Cardwell CR, Cantwell MM. (2013) Dietary fiber and the risk of precancerous lesions and cancer of the esophagus: a systematic review and meta-analysis. *Nutr Rev* **71**(7):474–82.

Cui L, Liu X, Tian Y, Xie C, Li Q, Cui H, Sun C. (2016) Flavonoids, flavonoid subclasses, and esophageal cancer risk: a meta-analysis of epidemiologic studies. *Nutrients* **8**(6):pii: E350.

Huang W, Han Y, Xu J, Zhu W, Li Z. (2013) Red and processed meat intake and risk of esophageal adenocarcinoma: a meta-analysis of observational studies. *Cancer Causes Control* **24**(1):193–201.

Islami F, Ren JS, Taylor PR, Kamangar F. (2009) Pickled vegetables and the risk of oesophageal cancer: a meta-analysis. *Br J Cancer* **101**(9):1641–7.

Jiang G, Li B, Liao X, Zhong C. (2016) Poultry and fish intake and risk of esophageal cancer: a meta-analysis of observational studies. *Asia Pac J Clin Oncol* **12**(1):e82–91.

Li B, Jiang G, Zhang G, Xue Q, Zhang H, Wang C, Zhao T. (2014) Intake of vegetables and fruit and risk of esophageal adenocarcinoma: a meta-analysis of observational studies. *Eur J Nutr* **53**(7):1511–21.

Liu J, Wang J, Leng Y, Lv C. (2013) Intake of fruit and vegetables and risk of esophageal squamous cell carcinoma: a meta-analysis of observational studies. *Int J Cancer* **133**(2):473–85.

Qu X, Ben Q, Jiang Y. (2013) Consumption of red and processed meat and risk for esophageal squamous cell carcinoma based on a meta-analysis, *Ann Epidemiol* **23**(12):762–70.

Salehi M, Moradi-Lakeh M, Salehi MH, Nojomi M, Kolahdooz F. (2013) Meat, fish, and esophageal cancer risk: a systematic review and dose-response meta-analysis. *Nutr Rev* **71**(5):257–67.

Sun L, Zhang Z, Xu J, Xu G, Liu X. (2017) Dietary fiber intake reduces risk for Barrett's esophagus and esophageal cancer. *Crit Rev Food Sci Nutr* **57**(13):2749–57.

Wang A, Zhu C, Fu L, Wan X, Yang X, Zhang H, Miao R, He L, Sang X, Zhao H. (2015) Citrus fruit intake substantially reduces the risk of esophageal cancer: a meta-analysis of epidemiologic studies. *Medicine (Baltimore)* **94**(39):e1390.

Zhao W, Liu L, Xu S. (2018) Intake of citrus fruit and risk of esophageal cancer: a meta-analysis. *Medicine (Baltimore)* **97**(13):e0018.

Zhu HC, Yang X, Xu LP, Zhao LJ, Tao GZ, Zhang C, Qin Q, Cai J, Ma JX, Mao WD, Zhang XZ, Cheng HY, Sun XC. (2014) Meat consumption is associated with esophageal cancer risk in a meat- and cancer-histological-type dependent manner. *Dig Dis Sci* **59**(3):664–73.

Heart disease

Afshin A, Micha R, Khatibzadeh S, Mozaffarian D. (2014) Consumption of nuts and legumes and risk incident ischemic heart disease, stroke, and diabetes: a systematic review and meta-analysis. *Am J Clin Nutr* **100**(1):278–88.

Bechthold A, Boeing H, Schwedhelm C, Hoffman G, Knuppel S, Iqbal K, De Henauw S, Michels N, Devleesschauwer B, Schlesinger S, Schwingshackl L. (2019) Food groups and risk of coronary heart disease, stroke and heart failure: a systematic review and dose-response meta-analysis of prospective studies. *Crit Rev Food Sci Nutr* **59**(7):1071–90.

Cui K, Liu Y, Zhu L, Mei X, Jin P, Luo Y. (2019) Association between intake of red and processed meat and the risk of heart failure: meta-analysis. *BMC Public Health* **19**(1):354.

Dinu M, Abbate R, Gensini GF, Casini A, Sofi F. (2017) Vegetarian, vegan diets and multiple health outcomes: a systematic review with meta-analysis of observational studies. *Crit Rev Food Sci Nutr* **57**(17):3640–9.

Gan Y, Tong X, Li L, Cao S, Yin X, Gao C, Herath C, Li W, Jin Z, Chen Y, Lu Z. (2015) Consumption of fruit and vegetable and risk of coronary heart disease: a meta-analysis of prospective cohort studies. *Int J Cardiol* **183**;129–37.

Graudal NA, Hubeck-Graudal T, Jurgens G. (2016) Reduced dietary sodium intake increases heart rate: a meta-analysis of 63 randomized controlled trials including 72 study populations. *Front Physiol* **7**:111.

He FJ, Nowson CA, Lucas M, MacGregor GA. (2007) Increased consumption of fruit and vegetables is related to a reduced risk of coronary heart disease: meta-analysis of cohort studies. *J Human Hypertens* **21**(9):717–28.

Huang C, Huang J, Tian Y, Yang X, Gu D. (2014) Sugar sweetened beverages consumption and risk of coronary heart disease: a meta-analysis of prospective studies. *Atherosclerosis* **234**(1):11–6.

Jiang W, Wei H, He B. (2015) Dietary flavonoids intake and the risk of coronary heart disease: a dose-response meta-analysis of 15 prospective studies. *Thromb Res* **135**(3):459–63.

Khawaja O, Singh H, Luni F, Kabour A, Ali SS, Taleb M, Ahmed H, Gaziano JM, Djousse L. (2017) Egg consumption and incidence of heart failure: a meta-analysis of prospective cohort studies. *Front Nutr* **4**:10.

Leung Yinko SS, Stark KD, Thanassoulis G, Pilote L. (2014) Fish consumption and acute coronary syndrome: a meta-analysis. *Am J Med* **127**(9):848–57.

Li YH, Zhou CH, Pei HJ, Zhou XL, Li LH, Wu YJ, Hui RT. (2013) Fish consumption and incidence of heart failure: a meta-analysis of prospective cohort studies. *Chin Med J (Engl)* **126**(5):942–8.

Lou D, Li Y, Yan G, Bu J, Wang H. (2016) Soy consumption with risk of coronary heart disease and stroke: the meta-analysis of observational studies. *Neuroepidemiology* **46**(4):242–52.

Ma L, Wang F, Guo W, Yang H, Liu Y, Zhang W. (2014) Nut consumption and the risk of coronary artery disease: a dose-response meta-analysis of 13 prospective studies. *Thromb Res* **134**(4):790–4.

Mahmassani HA, Avendano EE, Raman G, Johnson EJ. (2018) Avocado consumption and risk factors for heart disease: a systematic review and meta-analysis. *Am J Clin Nutr* **107**(4): 523–36.

Martinez-Gonzalez MA, Dominquez LJ, Delgado-Rodriguez M. (2014) Olive oil consumption and risk of CHD/or stroke: a meta-analysis of case-control, cohort and intervention studies. *Br J Nutr* **112**(2):248–59.

Mayr HL, Tierney AC, Thomas CJ, Ruiz-Canela M, Radcliffe J, Itsiopoulos C. (2018) Mediterranean-type diets and inflammatory markers in patients with coronary heart disease: a systematic review and meta-analysis. *Nutr Res* **50**:10–24.

Micha R, Wallace SK, Mozaffarian D. (2010) Red and processed meat consumption and risk of coronary heart disease, stroke, and diabetes mellitus: a systematic review and meta-analysis. *Circulation* **121**(21):2271–83.

Tang G, Wang D, Long J, Yang F, Si L. (2015) Meta-analysis of the association between whole grain intake and coronary heart disease risk. *Am J Cardiol* **115**(5):625–9.

Weng YQ, Yao J, Guo ML, Qin Qj, Li P. (2016) Association between nut consumption and coronary heart disease: a meta-analysis. *Coron Artery Dis* **27**(3):227–32.

Wu Y, Qian Y, Pan Y, Li P, Yang J, Ye X, Xu G. (2015) Association between dietary fiber intake and risk of coronary heart disease: a meta-analysis. *Clin Nutr* **34**(4):603–11.

Hypercholesterolemia (High blood cholesterol)

Anderson JW, Bush HM. (2011) Soy protein effects on serum lipoproteins: a quality assessment and meta-analysis of randomized, controlled studies. *J Am Coll Nutr* **30**(2):79–91.

Banel DK, Hu FB. (2009) Effects of walnut consumption on blood lipids and other cardiovascular risk factors: a meta-analysis and systematic review. *Am J Clin Nutr* **90**(1):56–63.

Bazzano LA, Thompson AM, Tees MT, Nguyen CH, Winham DM. (2011) Non-soy legume consumption lowers cholesterol levels: a meta-analysis of randomized controlled trials. *Nutr Metab Cardiovasc Dis* **21**(2):94–103

Chiavaroli L, de Souza RJ, Ha V, Cozma AI, Mirrahimi A, Wang DD, Yu M, Carleton AJ, Di Buono M, Jenkins AL, Leiter LA, Wolever TM, Beyene J, Kendall CW, Jenkins DJ, Sievenpiper JL. (2015) Effect of fructose on established lipid targets: a systematic review and meta-analysis of controlled feeding trials. *J Am Heart Assoc* 4(9):e001700.

De Goede J, Geleijnse JM, Ding EL, Soedamah-Muthu SS. (2015) Effect of cheese consumption on blood lipids: a systematic review and meta-analysis of randomized controlled trials. *Nutr Rev* 73(5):259–75.

Del Gobbo LC, Falk MC, Feldman R, Lewis K, Mozaffarian D. (2015) Effects of tree nuts on blood lipids, apolipoproteins, and blood pressure: systematic review, meta-analysis, and dose-response of 61 controlled intervention trials. *Am J Clin Nutr* 102(6):1347–56.

Ghobadi S, Hassanzadeh-Rostami Z, Mohammadian F, Nikfetrat A, Ghasemifard N, Raeisi Dehkordi H, Faghih S. (2018) Comparison of blood lipid-lowering effects of olive oil and other plant oils: a systematic review and meta-analysis of 27 randomized placebo-controlled clinical trials. *Crit Rev Food Sci Nutr* 8:1–15.

Harland JI, Haffner TA. (2008) Systematic review, meta-analysis and regression of randomized controlled trials reporting an association between an intake of circa 25 g soya protein per day and blood cholesterol. *Atherosclerosis* 200(1):13–27.

Hollander PL, Ross AB, Kristensen M. (2015) Whole-grain and blood lipid changes in apparently healthy adults: a systematic review and meta-analysis of randomized controlled studies. *Am J Clin Nutr* 102(3):556–72.

Jolfaie NR, Rouhani MH, Surkan PJ, Siassi F, Azadbakht L. (2016) Rice bran oil decreases total and LDL cholesterol in humans: a systematic review and meta-analysis of randomized controlled clinical trials. *Horm Metab Res* 48(7):417–26.

Kelishadi R, Mansourian M, Heidari-Beni M. (2014) Association of fructose consumption and components of metabolic syndrome in human studies: a systematic review and meta-analysis. *Nutrition* 30(5):503–10.

Mazidi M, Gao HK, Rezaie P, Ferns GA. (2016) The effect of ginger supplementation on serum C-reactive protein, lipid profile and glycaemia: a systematic review and meta-analysis. *Food Nutr Res* 60:32613.

Musa-Veloso K, Paulionis L, Poon T, Lee HY. (2016) The effects of almond consumption on fasting blood lipid levels: a systematic review and meta-analysis of randomized controlled trials. *J Nutr Sci* 5:e34.

Peou S, Milliard-Hasting B, Shah SA. (2016) Impact of avocado-enriched diets on plasma lipoproteins: a meta-analysis. *J Clin Lipidol* **10**(1):161–71.

Perna S, Giacosa A, Bonitta G, Bologna C, Isu A, Guido D, Rondanelli M. (2016) Effects of Hazelnut consumption on blood lipids and body weight: a systematic review and Bayesian meta-analysis. *Nutrients* **8**(12): pii: E747.

Ried K. (2016) Garlic lowers blood pressure in hypertensive individuals, regulates serum cholesterol, and stimulates immunity: An updated meta-analysis and review. *J Nutr* **146**(2):389S-396S.

Ried K, Toben C, Fakler P. (2013) Effect of garlic on serum lipids: an updated meta-analysis. *Nutr Rev* **71**(5):282–99.

Sabate J, Oda K, Ros E. (2010) Nut consumption and blood lipid levels: a pooled analysis of 25 intervention trials. *Arch Intern Med* **170**(9):821–7.

Simental-Mendia LE, Gotto AM Jr., Atkin SL, Banach M, Pirro M, Sahebkar A. (2018) Effect of soy isoflavone supplementation on plasma lipoprotein(a) concentrations: a meta-analysis. *J Clin Lipidol* **12**(1):16–24.

Sun Y, Neelakantan N, Wu Y, Lote-Oke R, Pan A, van Dam RM. (2015) Palm oil consumption increases LDL cholesterol compared with vegetable oils low in saturated fat in a meta-analysis of clinical trials. *J Nutr* **145**(7):1549–58

Tokede OA, Onabanjo TA, Yansane A, Gaziano JM, Djousse L. (2015) Soya products and serum lipids: a meta-analysis of randomized controlled trials. *Br J Nutr* **114**(6):831–43.

Wang F, Zheng J, Yang B, Jiang J, Fu Y, Li D. (2015) Effects of vegetarian diets on blood lipids: a systematic review and meta-analysis of randomized controlled trials. *J Am Heart Assoc* **4**(10):e002408.

Zeng T, Guo FF, Zhang CL, Song FY, Zhao XL, Xie KQ. (2012) A meta-analysis of randomized, double-blind, placebo-controlled trials for the effects of garlic on serum lipid profiles. *J Sci Food Agric* **92**(9):1892–902.

Zhang YH, An T, Zhang RC, Zhou Q, Huang Y, Zhang J. (2013) Very high fructose intake increases serum LDL-cholesterol and total cholesterol: a meta-analysis of controlled feeding trials. *J Nutr* **143**(9):1391–8.

Hypertension

Aburto NJ, Ziolkovska A, Hooper L, Elliot P, Cappuccino FP, Meerpohl JJ. (2013) Effect of lower sodium intake on health: Systemic review and meta-analysis. *BMJ* **346**:f1326

Cheungpasitporn W, Thongprayoon C, Edmonds PJ, Srivali N, Ungprasert P, Kittanamongkolchai W, Erickson SB. (2015) Sugar and artificially sweetened soda consumption linked to hypertension: a systematic review and meta-analysis. *Clin Exp Hypertens* **37**(7):587–93.

Dong JY, Tong X, Wu ZW, Xun PC, He K, Qin LQ. (2011) Effect of soya protein on blood pressure: a meta-analysis of randomized controlled trials. *Br J Nutr* **106**(3):317–26.

Evans CE, Greenwood DC, Threapleton DE, Cleghorn CL, Nykjaer C, Woodhead CE, Gale CP, Burley VJ. (2015) Effects of dietary fibre type on blood pressure: a systematic review and meta-analysis of randomized controlled trials of healthy individuals. *J Hypertens* **33**(5):897–911.

Fogacci F, Tocci G, Presta V, Fratter A, Borghi C, Cicero AFG. (2019) Effect of resveratrol on blood pressure: a systematic review and meta-analysis of randomized controlled, clinical trials. *Crit Rev Food Sci Nutr* **59**(10): 1605–18.

Graudal N, Hubeck-Graudal T, Jurgens G, McCarron DA. (2015) The significance of duration and amount of sodium reduction intervention in normotensive and hypertensive individuals: a meta-analysis. *Adv Nutr* **6**(2):169–77.

Guo K, Zhou Z, Jiang Y, Li W, Li Y. (2015) Meta-analysis of prospective studies on the effects of nut consumption on hypertensive and type 2 diabetes mellitus. *J Diabetes* **7**(2):202–12.

Ha V, Sievenpiper JL, de Souza RJ, Chiavaroli L, Wang DD, Cozma AI, Mirrahimi A, Yu ME, Carleton AJ, Dibuono M, Jenkins AL, Leiter LA, Wolever TM, Beyene J, Kendall CW, Jenkins DJ. (2012) Effect of fructose on blood pressure: a systematic review and meta-analysis of controlled feeding trials. *Hypertension* **59**(4):787–95.

He FJ, Li J, Macgregor GA. (2013) Effect of longer term modest salt reduction on blood pressure: Cochrane systematic review and meta-analysis of randomized trials. *BMJ* **346**:f1325.

Hidayat K, Du HZ, Yang J, Chen GC, Zhang Z, Li ZN, Qin LQ. (2017) Effects of milk proteins on blood pressure: a meta-analysis of randomized controlled trials. *Hypertens Res* **40**(3):264–70.

Jayalath VH, de Souza RJ, Ha V, Mirrahimi A, Blanco-Mejia S, Di Buono M, Jenkins AL, Leiter LA, Wolever TM, Beyene J, Kendall CW, Jenkins DJ, Sievenpiper JL. (2015) Sugar-sweetened beverage consumption and incident hypertension: a systematic review and meta-analysis of prospective cohorts. *Am J Clin Nutr* **102**(4):914–21.

Khalesi S, Irwin C, Schubert M. (2015) Flaxseed consumption may reduce blood pressure: a systematic review and meta-analysis of controlled trials. *J Nutr* **145**(4):758–65.

Li B, Li F, Wang L, Zhang D. (2016) Fruit and vegetables consumption and risk of hypertension: a meta-analysis. *J Clin Hypertens (Greenwich)* **18**(5):468–76.

Li SH, Zhao P, Tian HB, Chen LH, Cui LQ. (2015) Effect of grape polyphenols on blood pressure: a meta-analysis of randomized controlled trials. *PLoS One* **10**(9):e0137665.

Liu XX, Li SH, Chen JZ, Sun K, Wang XJ, Wang XG, Hui RT. (2012) Effect of soy isoflavones on blood pressure: a meta-analysis of randomized controlled trials. *Nutr Metab Cardiovasc Dis* **22**(6):463–70.

Liu Y, Ma W, Zhang P, He S, Huang D. (2015) Effect of resveratrol on blood pressure: a meta-analysis of randomized controlled trials. *Clin Nutr* **34**(1):27–34.

Lopez PD, Cativo FH, Atlas SA, Rosendorff C. (2019) The effect of vegan diets on blood pressure in adults: a meta-analysis of randomized controlled trials. *Am J Med* **132**(7):875–883.e7.

Mohammadifard N, Salehi-Abargouei A, Salas-Salvado J, Guasch-Ferre M, Humphries K, Sarrafzadegan N. (2015) The effect of tree nut, peanut, and soy nut consumption on blood pressure: a systematic review and meta-analysis of randomized controlled clinical trials. *Am J Clin Nutr* **101**(5):966–82.

Ralston RA, Lee JH, Truby H, Palermo CE, Walker KZ. (2012) A systematic review and meta-analysis of elevated blood pressure and consumption of dairy foods. *J Hum Hypertens* **26**(1):3–13.

Rebholz CM, Friedman EE, Powers LJ, Arroyave WD, He J, Kelly TN. (2012) Dietary protein intake and blood pressure: a meta-analysis of randomized controlled trials. *Am J Epidemiol* **176** Suppl 7:S27–43.

Sahebkar A, Ferri C, Giorgini P, Bo S, Nachtigal P, Grassi D. (2017) Effects of pomegranate juice on blood pressure: a systematic review and meta-analysis of randomized controlled trials. *Pharmacol Res* **115**:149–61.

Soedamah-Muthu SS, Verberne LD, Ding EL, Engberink MF, Geleijnse JM. (2012) Dairy consumption and incidence of hypertension: a dose-response meta-analysis of prospective cohort studies. *Hypertension* **60**(5):1131–7.

Taku K, Lin N, Cai D, Hu J, Zhao X, Zhang Y, Wang P, Melby MK, Hooper L, Kurzer MS, Mizuno S, Ishimi Y, Watanabe S. (2010) Effects of soy isoflavone extract supplements on blood pressure in adult humans: systematic review and meta-analysis of randomized placebo-controlled trials. *J Hypertens* **28**(10):1971–82.

Ursoniu S, Sahebkar A, Andrica F, Serban C, Banach M. (2016) Lipid and Blood Pressure Meta-analysis collaboration (LBPMC) group. Effects of flaxseed supplements on blood pressure: a systematic review and meta-analysis. *Clin Nutr* **35**(3):615–25.

Wang HP, Yang J, Qin LQ, Yang XJ. (2015) Effect of garlic on blood pressure: a meta-analysis. *J Clin Hypertens (Greenwich)* **17**(3):223–31.

Wang M, Moran AE, Liu J, Qi Y, Xie W, Tzong K, Zhao D. (2015) A meta-analysis of effect of dietary salt restriction on blood pressure in Chinese adults. *Glob Heart* **10**(4):291–9.

Wu L, Sun D, He Y. (2016) Fruit and vegetables consumption and incident hypertension: dose-response meta-analysis of prospective cohort studies. *J Hum Hypertens* **30**(10):573–80.

Xi B, Huang Y, Reilly KH, Li S, Zheng R, Barrio-Lopez MT, Martinez-Gonzalez MA, Zhou D. (2015) Sugar-sweetened beverages and risk of hypertension and CVD: a dose-response meta-analysis. *Br J Nutr* **113**(5):709–17.

Xiong XJ, Wang PQ, Li SJ, Li XK, Zhang YQ, Wang J. (2015) Garlic for hypertension: a systematic review and meta-analysis for randomized controlled trials. *Phytomedicine* **22**(3):352–61.

Yang B, Shi MQ, Li ZH, Yang JJ, Li D. (2016) Fish, long-chain n-3 PUFA and incidence of elevated blood pressure: a meta-analysis of prospective cohort studies. *Nutrients* **8**(1):pii: E58.

Zhang H, Liu S, Li L, Liu S, Liu S, Mi J, Tian G. (2016) The impact of grape seed extract treatment on blood pressure changes: a meta-analysis of 16 randomized controlled trials. *Medicine (Baltimore)* **95**(33):e4247.

Liver cancer

Gao M, Sun K, Guo M, Gao H, Liu K, Yang C, Li S, Liu N. (2015) Fish consumption and n-3 polyunsaturated fatty acids, and risk of hepatocellular carcinoma: a systematic review and meta-analysis. *Cancer Causes Control* **26**(3):367–76.

Huang YQ, Lu X, Min H, Wu QQ, Shi XT, Bian KQ, Zou XP. (2016) Green tea and liver cancer risk: the meta-analysis of prospective cohort studies in Asian populations. *Nutrition* **32**(1):3–8.

Luo AJ, Wang FZ, Luo D, Hu DH, Mao P, Xie WZ, He XF, Kan W, Wang Y. (2015) Consumption of vegetables may reduce the risk of liver cancer: results from the meta-analysis of case-control and cohort studies. *Clin Res Hepto-gastroenterol* **39**(1):45–51.

Luo J, Yang Y, Liu J, Lu K, Tang Z, Liu P, Liu L, Zhu Y. (2014) Systematic review with meta-analysis: meat consumption and the risk of hepatocellular carcinoma. *Aliment Pharmacol Ther* **39**(9):913–22.

Yang Y, Zhang D, Feng N, Chen G, Liu J, Chen G, Zhu Y. (2014) Increased intake of vegetables, but not fruit, reduces risk for hepatocellular carcinoma: a meta-analysis. *Gastroenterology* **147**(5):1031–42.

Lung cancer

Lippi G, Mattiuzzi C, Cervellin G. (2016) Meat consumption and cancer risk: a critical review of published meta-analyses. *Crit Rev Oncol Hematol* **97**:1–14.

Song J, Su H, Wang BL, Zhou YY, Guo LL. (2014) Fish consumption and lung cancer risk: systematic review and meta-analysis. *Nutr Cancer* **66**(4):539–49.

Sun Y, Li Z, Li J, Li Z, Han J. (2016) A healthy dietary pattern reduces lung cancer risk: a systematic review and meta-analysis. *Nutrients* **8**(3):134.

Tang NP, Zhou B, Wang B, Yu RB, Ma J. (2009) Flavonoids intake and risk of lung cancer: a meta-analysis. *Jpn J Clin Oncol* **39**(6):352–9.

Vieira AR, Abar L, Vingeliene S, Chan DS, Aune D, Navarro-Rosenblatt D, Stevens C, Greenwood D, Norat T. (2016) Fruits, vegetables and lung cancer risk: a systematic review and meta-analysis. *Ann Oncol* **27**(1):81–96.

Wakai K, Sugawara Y, Tsuji I, Tamakoshi A, Shimazu T, Matsuo K, Nagata C, Mizoue T, Tanaka K, Inoue M, Tsugane S, Sasazuki S. (2015) Research Group for the Development and Evaluation of Cancer Prevention Strategies in Japan. Risk of lung cancer and consumption of vegetables and fruit in Japanese: a pooled analysis of cohort studies in Japan. *Cancer Sci* **106**(8):1057–65.

Wang M, Qin S, Zhang T, Song X, Zhang S. (2015) The effect of fruit and vegetable intake on the development of lung cancer: a meta-analysis of 32 publications and 20,414 cases. *Eur J Clin Nutr* **69**(11):1184–92.

Wang Y, Li F, Wang Z, Qiu T, Shen T, Wang M. (2015) Fruit and vegetable consumption and risk of lung cancer: a dose-response meta-analysis of prospective cohort studies. *Lung Cancer* **88**(2):124–30.

Wu QJ, Xie L, Zheng W, Vogtmann E, Li HL, Yang G, Ji BT, Gao YT, Shu XO, Xiang YB. (2013) Cruciferous vegetables consumption and the risk of female lung cancer: a prospective study and a meta-analysis. *Ann Oncol* **24**(7):1918–24.

Wu SH, Liu Z. (2013) Soy food consumption and lung cancer risk: a meta-analysis using a common measure across studies. *Nutr Cancer.* **65**(5):625–32.

Xue XJ, Gao Q, Qiao JH, Zhang J, Xu CP, Liu J. (2014) Red and processed meat consumption and the risk of lung cancer: a dose-response meta-analysis of 33 published studies. *Int J Clin Exp Med* **7**(6):1542–53.

Xue Y, Jiang Y, Jin S, Li Y. (2016) Association between cooking oil fume exposure and lung cancer among Chinese nonsmoking women: a meta-analysis. *Onco Targets Ther* **9**:2987–92.

Yang G, Shu XO, Chow WH, Zhang X, Li HL, Ji BT, Cai H, Wu S, Gao YT, Zheng W. (2012) Soy food intake and risk of lung cancer: evidence from the Shanghai Women's Health Study and a meta-analysis. *Am J Epidemiol* **176**(10):846–55.

Yang WS, Va P, Wong MY, Zhang HL, Xiang YB. (2011) Soy intake is associated with lower lung cancer risk: results from a meta-analysis of epidemiologic studies. *Am J Clin Nutr* **94**(6):1575–83.

Yang WS, Wong MY, Vogtmann E, Tang RQ, Xie L, Yang YS, Wu QJ, Zhang W, Xiang YB. (2012) Meat consumption and risk of lung cancer: evidence from observational studies. *Ann Oncol* **23**(12):3163–70.

Obesity

Andela S, Burrows TL, Baur LA, Coyle DH, Collins CE, Gow ML. (2019) Efficacy of very low-energy diet programs for weight loss: a systematic review with meta-analysis of intervention studies in children and adolescents with obesity. *Obes Rev* **20**(6):871–82.

Abargouei AS, Janghorbani M, Salehi-Mazijarani M, Esmaillzadeh A. (2012) Effect of dairy consumption on weight and body composition in adults: a systematic review and meta-analysis of randomized controlled trials. *Int J Obes.* (Lond) **36**(12):1485–93.

Barnard ND, Levin SM, Yokoyama Y. (2015) A systematic review and meta-analysis of changes in body weight in clinical trials of vegetarian diets. *J Acad Nutr Diet* **115**(6):954–69.

Bertoia ML, Mukamal KJ, Cahill LE, Hou T, Ludwig DS, Mozaffarian D, Willett WC, Hu FB, Rimm EB. (2015) Changes in intake of fruits and vegetables and weight change in United States men and women followed for up to 24 years: analysis from three prospective cohort studies. *PLoS Med* **12**(9):e1001878.

Brunkwall L, Chen Y, Hindy G, Rukh G, Ericson U, Barroso I, Johansson I, Franks PW, Orho-Melander M, Renstrom F. (2016) Sugar-sweetened beverage consumption and genetic predisposition to obesity in 2 Swedish cohorts. *Am J Clin Nutr* **104**(3):809–15.

Chen M, Pan A, Malik VS, Hu FB. (2012) Effects of dairy intake on body weight and fat: a meta-analysis of randomized controlled trials. *Am J Clin Nutr* **96**(4):735–47.

Chiavaroli L, Kendall CWC, Braunstein CR, Blanco Mejia S, Leiter LA, Jenkins DJA, Sievenpiper JL. (2018) Effect of pasta in the context of low-glycemic index dietary patterns on body weight and markers of adiposity: a systematic review and meta-analysis of randomized controlled trials in adults. *BMJ Open* **8**(3):e019438.

Hashimoto Y, Fukuda T, Oyabu C, Tanaka M, Asano M, Yamazaki M, Fukui M. (2016) Impact of low-carbohydrate diet on body composition:

meta-analysis of randomized controlled studies. *Obes Rev* **17**(6): 499–509.

Huang RY, Huang CC, Hu FB, Chavarro JE. (2016) Vegetarian diets and weight reduction: a meta-analysis of randomized controlled trials. *J Gen Intern Med* **31**(1):109–16.

Jiao J, Xu JY, Zhang W, Han S, Qin LQ. (2015) Effect of dietary fiber on circulating C-reactive protein in overweight and obese adults: a meta-analysis of randomized controlled trials. *Int J Food Sci Nutr* **66**(1):114–9.

Kim SJ, de Sourza RJ, Choo VL, Ha V, Cozma AI, Chiavaroli L, Mirrahimi A, Blanco Mejia S, Di Buono M, Berstein AM, Leiter LA, Kris-Etherton PM, Vuksan V, Beyene J, Kendall CW, Jenkins DJ, Sievenpiper JL. (2016) Effects of dietary pulse consumption on body weight: a systematic review and meta-analysis of randomized controlled trials. *Am J Clin Nutr* **103**(5):1213–23.

Lu L, Xun P, Wan Y, He K, Cai W. (2016) Long-term association between dairy consumption and risk of childhood obesity: a systematic review and meta-analysis of prospective cohort studies. *Eur J Clin Nutr* **70**(4):414–23.

Malik VS, Pan A, Willett WC, Hu FB. (2013) Sugar-sweetened beverages and weight gain in children and adults: a systematic review and meta-analysis. *Am J Clin Nutr* **98**(4):1084–102.

Mytton OT, Nnoaham K, Eyles H, Scarborough P, Ni Mhurchu C. (2014) Systematic review and meta-analysis of the effect of increased vegetable and fruit consumption on body weight and energy intake. *BMC Public Health* **14**:886.

Rahmani J, Miri A, Cerneviciute R, Thompson J, de Souza NN, Sultana R, Kord Varkaneh H, Mousavi SM, Hekmatdoost A. (2019) Effects of cereal beta-glucan consumption on body weight, body mass index, waist circumference, and total energy intake: a meta-analysis of randomized controlled trials. *Complement Ther Med* **43**:131–9.

Rouhani MH, Haghighatdoost F, Surkan PJ, Azadbakht L. (2016) Associations between dietary energy density and obesity: a systematic review and meta-analysis of observational studies. *Nutrition* **32**(10):1037–47.

Ruanpeng D, Thongprayoon C, Cheungpasitporn W, Harindhanavudhi T. (2017) Sugar and artificially-sweetened beverages linked to obesity: a systematic review and meta-analysis. *QJM* **110**(8):513–20.

Stelmach-Mardas M, Rodacki T, Dobrowolska-Iwanek J, Brzozowska A, Walkowiak J, Wojtanowska-Krosniak A, Zagrodzki P, Bechthold A, Mardas M, Boeing H. (2016) Link between food energy density and body weight changes in obese adults. *Nutrients* **8**(4):229.

Stelmach-Mardas M, Walkowiak J. (2016) Dietary interventions and changes in cardio-metabolic parameters in metabolically healthy obese subjects: a systematic review with meta-analysis. *Nutrients* **8**(8):pii: E455.

Sievenpiper JL, de Souza RJ, Mirrahimi A, Yu ME, Carleton AJ, Beyene K, Chiavaroli L, Di Buono M, Jenkins AL, Leiter LA, Wolever TM, Kendall CW, Jenkins DJ. (2012) Effect of fructose on body weight in controlled feeding trials: a systematic review and meta-analysis. *Ann Intern Med* **156**(4):291–304.

Verheggen RJ, Maessen MF, Green DJ, Hermus AR, Hopman MT, Thijssen DH. (2016) A systematic review and meta-analysis on the effects of exercise training versus hypocaloric diet: distinct effects on body weight and visceral adipose tissue. *Obes Rev* **17**(8):664–90.

Wang W, Wu Y, Zhang D. (2016) Association of dairy products consumption with risk of obesity in children and adults: a meta-analysis of mainly cross-sectional studies. *Ann Epidemiol* **26**(12):870–82.

Ye EQ, Chacko SA, Chou EL, Kugizaki M, Liu S. (2012) Greater whole-grain intake is associated with lower risk of type 2 diabetes, cardiovascular disease, and weight gain. *J Nutr* **142**(7):1304–13.

Zhang YB, Chen WH, Guo JJ, Fu ZH, Yi C, Zhang M, Na XL. (2013) Soy isoflavone supplementation could reduce body weight and improve glucose metabolism in non-Asian postmenopausal women-a meta-analysis. *Nutrition* **29**(1):8–14.

Zibellini J, Seimon RV, Lee CM, Gibson AA, Hsu MS, Sainsbury A. (2016) Effect of diet-induced weight loss on muscle strength in adults with overweight or obesity — a systematic review and meta-analysis of clinical trials. *Obes Rev* **17**(8):647–63.

Oral cancer

Aminianfar A, Fallah-Moshkani R, Salari-Moghaddam A, Saneei P, Larijani B, Esmailzadeh A. (2019) Egg consumption and risk of upper aero-digestive tract cancers: a systematic review and meta-analysis of observational studies. *Adv Nutr* 10(4):660–72.

Edefonti V, Hashibe M, Parpinel M, Turati F, Serraino D, Matsuo K, Olshan AF, Zevallos JP, Winn DM, Moysich K, Zhang ZF, Morgenstern H, Levi F, Kelsey K, McClean M, Bosetti C, Galeone C, Schantz S, Yu GP, Boffetta P, Amy Lee YC, Chuang SC, La Vecchia C, Decarli A. (2015) Natural vitamin C intake and the risk of head and neck cancer: a pooled analysis in the International Head and Neck Cancer Epidemiology Consortium. *Int J Cancer* 137(2):448–62.

Guha N, Warnakulasuriya S, Vlaanderen J, Straif K. (2014) Betel quid chewing and the risk of oral and oropharyngeal cancers: a meta-analysis with implications for cancer control. *Int J Cancer* 135(6):1433–43.

Gupta B, Johnson NW. (2014) Systematic review and meta-analysis of association between smokeless tobacco and of betel quid without tobacco with incidence of oral cancer in South Asia and the Pacific. *PLoS One* 9(11):e113385.

Pavia M, Pileggi C, Nobile CG, Angelillo IF. (2016) Association between fruit and vegetable consumption and oral cancer: a meta-analysis of observational studies. *Am J Clin Nutr* 83(5):1126–34.

Petti S, Masood M, Scully C. (2013) The magnitude of tobacco smoking — betel quid chewing — alcohol drinking interaction effect on oral cancer in South-East Asia: a meta-analysis of observational studies. *PLoS One* 8(11):e78999.

Ovarian cancer

Han B, Li X, Yu T. (2014) Cruciferous vegetables consumption and the risk of ovarian cancer: a meta-analysis of observational studies. *Diagn Pathol* 9:7.

Hu J, Hu Y, Hu Y, Zheng S. (2015) Intake of cruciferous vegetables is associated with reduced risk of ovarian cancer: a meta-analysis. *Asia Pac J Clin Nutr* 24(1):101–9.

Hua X, Yu L, You R, Yang Y, Liao J, Chen D, Yu L. (2016) Association among dietary flavonoids, flavonoid subclasses and ovarian cancer risk: a meta-analysis. *PLoS One* 11(3):e0151134.

Huang X, Wang X, Shang J, Lin Y, Yang Y, Song Y, Yu S. (2018) Association between dietary fiber intake and risk of ovarian cancer: a meta-analysis of observational studies. *J Int Med Res* **46**(10):3995–4005.

Huncharek M, Kupelnick B. (2001) Dietary fat intake and risk of epithelial ovarian cancer: a meta-analysis of 6,689 subjects from 8 observational studies. *Nutr Cancer* **40**(2):87–91.

Kolahdooz F, van der Pols JC, Bain CJ, Marks GC, Hughes MC, Whiteman DC, Webb PM. (2010) Australian Cancer Study (Ovarian Cancer) and the Australian Ovarian Cancer Study Group. Meat, fish, and ovarian cancer risk: results from 2 Australian case-control studies, a systematic review, and meta-analysis. *Am J Clin Nutr* **91**(6):1752–63.

Merritt MA, Tzoulaki I, van den Brandt PA, Schouten LJ, Tsilidis KK, Weiderpass E, Patel CJ, Tionneland A, Hansen L, Overvad K, His M, Dartois L, Boutron-Ruault MC, Fortner RT, Kaaks R, Aleksandrova K, Boeing H, Trichopoulou A, Lagiou P, Bamia C, Palli D, Krogh V, Tumino R, Ricceri F, Mattiello A, Bueno-de-Mesquita HB, Onland-Moret NC, Peeters PH, Skeie G, Jareid M, Quiros JR, Obon-Santacana M, Sanchez MJ, Chamosa S, Huerta JM, Barricarte A, Dias JA, Sonestedt E, Idahl A, Lundin E, Wareham NJ, Khaw KT, Travis RC, Ferrari P, Riboli E, Gunter MJ. (2016) Nutrient-wide association study of 57 foods/nutrients and epithelial ovarian cancer in the European prospective investigation into cancer and nutrition study and the Netherlands cohort study. *Am J Clin Nutr* **103**(1):161–7.

Qu XL, Fang Y, Zhang M, Zhang YZ. (2014) Phytoestrogen intake and risk of ovarian cancer: a meta-analysis of 10 observational studies. *Asian Pac J Cancer Prev* **15**(21):9085–91.

Zeng ST, Guo L, Liu SK, Wang DH, Xi J, Huang P, Liu DT, Gao JF, Feng J, Zhang L. (2015) Egg consumption is associated with increased risk of ovarian cancer: evidence from a meta-analysis of observational studies. *Clin Nutr* **34**(4):635–41.

Pancreatic cancer

Bae JM, Lee EJ, Guyatt G. (2009) Citrus fruit intake and pancreatic cancer risk: a quantitative systematic review. *Pancreas* **38**(2):168–74.

Larsson SC, Wolk A. (2012) Red and processed meat consumption and risk of pancreatic cancer: meta-analysis of prospective studies. *Br J Cancer* **106**(3):603–7.

Lei Q, Zheng H, Bi J, Wang X, Jiang T, Gao X, Tian F, Xu M, Wu C, Zhang L, Li N, Li J. (2016) Whole grain intake reduces pancreatic cancer risk: the meta-analysis of observational studies. *Medicine (Baltimore)* **95**(9):e2747.

Li LY, Luo Y, Lu MD, Xu XW, Lin HD, Zheng ZQ. (2015) Cruciferous vegetable consumption and the risk of pancreatic cancer: a meta-analysis. *World J Surg Oncol* **13**:44.

Mao QQ, Lin YW, Chen H, Qin J, Zheng XY, Xu X, Xie LP. (2017) Dietary fiber intake is inversely associated with risk of pancreatic cancer: a meta-analysis. *Asian Pac J Clin Nutr* **26**(1):89–96.

Paluszkiewicz P, Smolinska K, Debinska I, Turski WA. (2012) Main dietary compounds and pancreatic cancer risk: the quantitative analysis of case control and cohort studies. *Cancer Epidemiol* **36**(1):60–7.

Wang CH, Qian C, Wang RC, Zhou WP. (2015) Dietary fiber intake and pancreatic cancer risk: a meta-analysis of epidemiological studies. *Sci Rep* **5**:10834.

Zhao Z, Yin Z, Pu Z, Zhao Q. (2017) Association between consumption of red and processed meat and pancreatic cancer risk: a systematic review and meta-analysis. *Clin Gastroenterol Hepatol* **15**(4):486–93.

Premature mortality

Abete I, Romaguera D, Vieira AR, Lopez de Munain A, Norat T. (2014) Association between total, processed, red and white meat consumption and all-cause, CVD and IHD mortality: a meta-analysis of cohort studies. *Br J Nutr* **112**(5):762–75.

Aune D, Giovannucci E, Boffetta P, Fadnes LT, Keum N, Norat T, Greenwood DC, Riboli E, Vatten LJ, Tonstad S. (2017) Fruit and vegetable intake and the risk of cardiovascular disease, total cancer and all-cause mortality — a systematic review and dose-response meta-analysis of prospective studies. *Int J Epidemiol* **46**(3):1029–56.

Aune D, Keum N, Giovannucci E, Fadnes LT, Boffetta P, Greenwood DC, Tonstad S, Vatten LJ, Riboli E, Norat T. (2016) Nut consumption and risk of cardiovascular disease, total cancer, all-cause and cause-specific mortality: a systematic review and dose-response meta-analysis of prospective studies. *BMC Med* **14**(1):207.

Benisi-Kohansal S, Saneei P, Salehi-Marzijarani M, Larijani B, Esmaillzadeh A. (2016) Whole-grain intake and mortality from all causes, cardiovascular disease, and cancer: a systematic review and dose-response meta-analysis of prospective cohort studies. *Adv Nutr* **7**(6):1052–65.

Chen GC, Tong X, Xu JY, Han SF, Wan ZX, Qin JB, Qin LQ. (2016) Whole-grain intake and total, cardiovascular, and cancer mortality: a systematic review and meta-analysis of prospective studies. *Am J Clin Nutr* **104**(1):164–72.

Graudal N, Jurgens G, Baslund B, Alderman MH. (2014) Compared with usual sodium intake, low- and excessive-sodium diets are associated with increased mortality: a meta-analysis. *Am J Hypertens* **27**(9): 1129–37.

Grosso G, Yang J, Marventano S, Micek A, Galvano F, Kales SN. (2015) Nut consumption on all-cause, cardiovascular, and cancer mortality risk: a systematic review and meta-analysis of epidemiologic studies. *Am J Clin Nutr* **101**(4):783–93.

Hajishafiee M, Saneei P, Benisi-Kohansal S, Esmaillzadeh A. (2016) Cereal fibre intake and risk of mortality from all causes, CVD, cancer and inflammatory disease: a systematic review and meta-analysis prospective cohort studies. *Br J Nutr* **116**(2):343–52.

He J, Gu Y, Zhang S. (2017) Consumption of vegetables and fruits and breast cancer survival: a systematic review and meta-analysis. *Sci Rep* **7**(1):599.

Kelly JT, Palmer SC, Wai SN, Ruospo M, Carrero JJ, Campbell KL, Strippoli GF. (2017) Healthy dietary patterns and risk of mortality and ESRD in CKD: a meta-analysis of cohort studies. *Clin J Am Soc Nephrol* **12**(2):272–9.

Kim Y, Je Y. (2016) Dietary fibre intake and mortality from cardiovascular disease and all cancers: a meta-analysis of prospective cohort studies. *Arch Cardiovasc Dis* **109**(1):39–54.

Kim Y, Je Y. (2014) Dietary fiber intake and total mortality: a meta-analysis of prospective cohort studies. *Am J Epidemiol* **180**(6): 565–73.

Larsson SC, Orsini N. (2104) Red meat and processed meat consumption and all-cause mortality: a meta-analysis. *Am J Epidemiol* **179**(3):282–9.

Li B, Zhang G, Tan M, Zhao L, Jin L, Tang X, Jiang G, Zhong K. (2016) Consumption of whole grains in relation to mortality from all causes, cardiovascular disease, and diabetes: dose-response meta-analysis of prospective cohort studies. *Medicine (Baltimore)* **95**(33):e4229.

Liu L, Wang S, Liu J. (2015) Fiber consumption and all-cause, cardiovascular, and cancer mortality: a systematic review and meta-analysis of cohort studies. *Mol Nutr Food Res* **59**(1):139–46.

Liu XM, Liu YJ, Huang Y, Yu HJ, Yuan S, Tang BW, Wang PG, He QQ. (2017) Dietary total flavonoids intake and risk of mortality from all causes and cardiovascular disease in the general population: a systematic review and meta-analysis of cohort studies. *Mol Nutr Food Res* **61**(6):1601003.

Lu W, Chen H, Niu Y, Wu H, Xia D, Wu Y. (2016) Dairy products intake and cancer mortality risk: a meta-analysis of 11 population-based cohort studies. *Nutr J* **15**(1):91.

Ma X, Tang WG, Yang Y, Zhang QL, Zheng JL, Xiang YB. (2016) Association between whole grain intake and all-cause mortality: a meta-analysis of cohort studies. *Oncotarget* **7**(38):61996–62005.

Micha R, Penalvo JL, Cudhea F, Imamura F, Rehm CD, Mozaffarian D. (2017) Association between dietary factors and mortality from heart disease, stroke and type 2 diabetes in the United States. *JAMA* **317**(9):912–24.

Nachvak SM, Moradi S, Anjom-Shoae J, Rahmani J, Nasiri J, Maleki V, Sadeghi O. (2019) Soy, soy isoflavones, and protein intake in relation to mortality from all causes, cancers, and cardiovascular diseases: a systematic review and dose-response meta-analysis of prospective cohort studies. *J Acad Nutr Diet* **119**(9):1483–1500.

Onvani S, Haghighatdoost F, Surkan PJ, Larijani B, Azadbakht L. (2017) Adherence to the healthy eating index and alternative healthy eating index dietary patterns and mortality from all causes, cardiovascular disease and cancer: the meta-analysis of observational studies. *J Hum Nutr Diet* **30**(2):216–26.

Poggio R, Gutierrez L, Matta MG, Elorriaga N, Irazola V, Rubinstein A. (2015) Daily sodium consumption and CVD mortality in the general population: systematic review and meta-analysis of prospective studies. *Public Health Nutr* **18**(4):695–704.

Saneei P, Larijani B, Esmaillzadeh A. (2017) Rice consumption, incidence of chronic diseases and risk of mortality: meta-analysis of cohort studies. *Public Health Nutr* **20**(2):233–44.

Schwedhelm C, Boeing H, Hoffmann G, Aleksandrova K, Schwingshackl L. (2016) Effect of diet on mortality and cancer recurrence among cancer survivors: a systematic review and meta-analysis of cohort studies. *Nutr Rev* **74**(12):737–48.

Schwingshackl L, Hoffmann G. (2014) Monounsaturated fatty acids, olive oil and health status: a systematic review and meta-analysis of cohort studies. *Lipids Health Dis* **13**:154.

Schwingshackl L, Schwedhelm C, Hoffmann G, Lampousi AM, Knuppel S, Iqbal K, Bechthold A, Schlesinger S, Boeing H. (2017) Food groups and risk of all-cause mortality: a systematic review and meta-analysis of prospective studies. *Am J Clin Nutr* **105**(6):1462–73.

Van den Brandt PA, Schouten LJ. (2015) Relationship of tree nut, peanut and peanut butter intake with total and cause-specific mortality: a cohort study and meta-analysis. *Int J Epidemiol* **44**(3):1038–49.

Wang X, Lin X, Ouyang YY, Liu J, Zhao G, Pan A, Hu FB. (2016) Red and processed meat consumption and mortality: dose-response meta-analysis of prospective cohort studies. *Public Health Nutr* **19**(5):893–905.

Wang X, Ouyang Y, Liu J, Zhu M, Zhao G, Bao W, Hu FB. (2014) Fruit and vegetable consumption and mortality from all causes, cardiovascular disease, and cancer: systematic review and dose-response meta-analysis of prospective cohort studies. *BMJ* **349**:g4490.

Wei H, Gao Z, Liang R, Li Z, Hao H, Liu X. (2016) Whole-grain consumption and the risk of all-cause, CVD and cancer mortality: a meta-analysis of prospective cohort studies. *Br J Nutr* **116**(3):514–25.

Yamada T, Hara K, Kadowaki T. (2013) Chewing betel quid and the risk of metabolic disease, cardiovascular disease, and all-cause mortality: a meta-analysis. *PLoS One* **8**(8):e70679.

Yang Y, Zhao LG, Wu QJ, Ma X, Xiang YB. (2015) Association between dietary fiber and lower risk of all-cause mortality: a meta-analysis of cohort studies. *Am J Epidemiol* **181**(2):83–91.

Zhang B, Zhao Q, Guo W, Bao W, Wang X. (2018) Association of whole grain intake with all-cause, cardiovascular, and cancer mortality: a systematic review and dose-response meta-analysis from prospective cohort studies. *Eur J Clin Nutr* 72(1):57–65.

Zhao LG, Sun JW, Yang Y, Ma X, Wang YY, Xiang YB. (2016) Fish consumption and all-cause mortality: a meta-analysis of cohort studies. *Eur J Clin Nutr* 70(2):155–61.

Zheng J, Huang T, Yu Y, Hu X, Yang B, Li D. (2012) Fish consumption and CHD mortality: an updated meta-analysis of seventeen cohort studies. *Public Health Nutr* 15(4):725–37.

Zong G, Gao A, Hu FB, Sun Q. (2016) Whole grain intake and mortality from all causes, cardiovascular disease, and cancer: a meta-analysis of prospective cohort studies. *Circulation* 133(24):2370–80.

Prostate cancer

Applegate CC, Rowles JL, Ranard KM, Jeon S, Erdman JW. (2018) Soy consumption and risk of prostate cancer: an updated systematic review and meta-analysis. *Nutrients* 10(1):E40.

Chen J, Song Y, Zhang L. (2013) Lycopene/tomato consumption and the risk of prostate cancer: a systematic review and meta-analysis of prospective studies. *J Nutr Sci Vitaminol (Tokyo)* 59(3):213–23.

Chen P, Zhang W, Wang X, Zhao K, Negi DS, Zhuo L, Qi M, Wang X, Zhang X. (2015) Lycopene and risk of prostate cancer: a systematic review and meta-analysis. *Medicine (Baltimore)* 94(33):e1260.

Etminan M, Takkouche B, Caamano-Isorna F. (2004) The role of tomato products and lycopene in the prevention of prostate cancer: a meta-analysis of observational studies. *Cancer Epidemiol Biomarkers Prev* 13(3):340–5.

Fabiani R, Minelli L, Bertarelli G, Bacci S. (2016) A western dietary pattern increases prostate cancer risk: a systematic review and meta-analysis. *Nutrients* 8(10):pii: E626.

Godos J, Bella F, Sciacca S, Galvano F, Grosso G. (2017) Vegetarianism and breast, colorectal and prostate cancer risk: an overview and meta-analysis of cohort studies. *J Hum Nutr Diet* 30(3):349–59.

Harrison S, Lennon R, Holly J, Higgins JP, Gardner M, Perks C, Gaunt T, Tan V, Borwick C, Emmet P, Jeffreys M, Northstone K, Rinaldi S, Thomas S, Turner SD, Pease A, Vilenchick V, Martin RM, Lewis SJ. (2017) Does milk intake promote prostate cancer initiation or progression via effects on insulin-like growth factor (IGFs)? A systematic review and meta-analysis. *Cancer Causes Control* 28(6):497–528.

Hwang YW, Kim SY, Jee SH, Kim YN, Nam CM. (2009) Soy food consumption and risk of prostate cancer: a meta-analysis of observational studies. *Nutr Cancer* 61(5):598–606.

Li J, Mao QQ. (2017) Legume intake and risk of prostate cancer: a meta-analysis of prospective cohort studies. *Oncotarget* 8(27):44776–84.

Lippi G, Mattiuzzi C. (2015) Fried food and prostate cancer risk: systematic review and meta-analysis. *Int J Food Sci Nutr* 66(5):587–9.

Liu B, Mao Q, Cao M, Xie L. (2012) Cruciferous vegetables intake and risk of prostate cancer: a meta-analysis. *Int J Urol* 19(2):134–41.

Mohseni R, Abbasi S, Mohseni F, Rahimi F, Alizadeh S. (2019) Association between dietary inflammatory index and the risk of prostate cancer: a meta-analysis. *Nutr Cancer* 71(3):359–66.

Rowles JL 3rd, Ranard KM, Applegate CC, Jeon S, An R, Erdman JW Jr. (2018) Processed and raw tomato consumption and risk of prostate cancer: a systematic review and dose-response meta-analysis. *Prostate Cancer Prostatic Dis* 21(3):319–36.

Szymanski KM, Wheeler DC, Mucci LA. (2010) Fish consumption and prostate cancer risk: a review and meta-analysis. *Am J Clin Nutr* 92(5):1223–33.

Van Die MD, Bone KM, Williams SG, Pirotta MV. (2014) Soy and soy isoflavones in prostate cancer: a systematic review and meta-analysis of randomized controlled trials. *BJU Int* 113(5b):E119–30.

Xu X, Li J, Wang X, Wang S, Meng S, Zhu Y, Liang Z, Zheng X, Xie L. (2016) Tomato consumption and prostate cancer risk: a systematic review and meta-analysis. *Sci Rep* 6:37091.

Yan L, Spitznagel EL. (2009) Soy consumption and prostate cancer risk in men: a revisit of the meta-analysis. *Am J Clin Nutr* 89(4):1155–63.

Zhou XF, Ding ZS, Liu NB. (2013) Allium vegetables and risk of prostate cancer: evidence from 132,192 subjects. *Asian Pac J Cancer Prev* 14(7):4131–4.

Stomach cancer

Bae JM, Kim EH. (2016) Dietary intakes of citrus fruit and risk of gastric cancer incidence: an adaptive meta-analysis of cohort studies. *Epidemiol Health* **38**:e2016034.

Bertuccio P, Rosato V, Andreano A, Ferraroni M, Decarli A, Edefonti V, La Vecchia C. (2013) Dietary patterns and gastric cancer risk: a systematic review and meta-analysis. *Ann Oncol* **24**(6):1450–8.

D'Elia L, Rossi G, Ippolito R, Cappuccio FP, Strazzullo P. (2012) Habitual salt intake and risk of gastric cancer: a meta-analysis of prospective studies. *Clin Nutr* **31**(4):489–98.

Fallahzadeh H, Jalali A, Momayyezi M, Bazm S. (2015) Effect of carrot intake in the prevention of gastric cancer: a meta-analysis. *J Gastric Cancer* **15**(4):256–61.

Fang X, Wei J, He X, An P, Wang H, Jiang L, Shao D, Liang H, Li Y, Wang F, Min J. (2015) Landscape of dietary factors associated with risk of gastric cancer: a systematic review and dose-response meta-analysis of prospective cohort studies. *Eur J Cancer* **51**(18):2820–32.

Ge S, Feng X, Shen L, Wei Z, Zhu Q, Sun J. (2012) Association between habitual dietary salt intake and risk of gastric cancer: a systematic review of observational studies. *Gastroenterol Res Pract* **2012**:808120.

Kim HJ, Lim SY, Lee JS, Park S, Shin A, Choi BY, Shimazu T, Inoue M, Tsugane S, Kim J. (2010) Fresh and pickled vegetable consumption and gastric cancer in Japanese and Korean populations: a meta-analysis of observational studies. *Cancer Sci* **101**(2):508–16.

Kim J, Kang M, Lee JS, Inoue M, Sasazuki S, Tsugane S. (2011) Fermented and non-fermented soy food consumption and gastric cancer in Japanese and Korean populations: a meta-analysis of observational studies. *Cancer Sci* **102**(1):231–44.

Kodali RT, Eslick GD. (2015) Meta-analysis: does garlic intake reduce risk of gastric cancer? *Nutr Cancer* **67**(1):1–11.

Lu D, Pan C, Ye C, Duan H, Xu F, Yin L, Tian W, Zhang S. (2017) Meta-analysis of soy consumption and gastrointestinal cancer risk. *Sci Rep* **7**(1):4048.

Mahjub H, Sadri G. (2007) Association between alcohol consumption and gastric cancer: a meta-analysis. *J Res Health Sci* **7**(2):63–72.

Ren JS, Kamangar F, Forman D, Islami F. (2012) Pickled food and risk of gastric cancer — a systematic review and meta-analysis of English and Chinese literature. *Cancer Epidemiol Biomarkers Prev* **21**(6):905–15.

Shimazu T, Wakai K, Tamakoshi A, Tsuji I, Tanaka K, Matsuo K, Nagata C, Mizoue T, Inoue M, Tsugane S, Sazazuki A. (2014) Research Group for the Development and Evaluation of Cancer Prevention Strategies in Japan. Association of vegetable and fruit intake with gastric cancer risk among Japanese: a pooled analysis of four cohort studies. *Ann Oncol* **25**(6):1228–33.

Song P, Lu M, Yin Q, Wu L, Zhang D, Fu B, Wang B, Zhao Q. (2014) Red meat consumption and stomach cancer risk: a meta-analysis. *J Cancer Res Clin Oncol* **140**(6):979–92.

Turati F, Pelucchi C, Guercio V, La Vecchia C, Galeone C. (2015) Allium vegetable intake and gastric cancer: a case-control study and meta-analysis. *Mol Nutr Food Res* **59**(1):171–9.

Wang Q, Chen Y, Wang X, Gong G, Li G, Li C. (2014) Consumption of fruit, but not vegetables, may reduce risk of gastric cancer: results from the meta-analysis of cohort studies. *Eur J Cancer* **50**(8):1498–509.

Woo HD, Park S, Oh K, Kim HJ, Shin HR, Moon HK, Kim J. (2014) Diet and cancer risk in the Korean population: a meta-analysis. *Asian Pac J Cancer Prev* **15**(19):8509–19.

Wu QJ, Yang Y, Wang J, Han LH, Xiang YB. (2013) Cruciferous vegetable consumption and gastric cancer risk: a meta-analysis of epidemiological studies. *Cancer Sci* **104**(8):1067–73.

Xie Y, Huang S, Su Y. (2016) Dietary flavonols intake and risk of esophageal and gastric cancer: a meta-analysis of epidemiological studies. *Nutrients* **8**(2):91.

Yang T, Yang X, Wang X, Wang Y, Song Z. (2013) The role of tomato products and lycopene in the prevention of gastric cancer: a meta-analysis of epidemiologic studies. *Med Hypotheses* **80**(4):383–8.

Zhang Z, Xu G, Ma M, Yang J, Liu X. (2013) Dietary fiber intake reduces risk for gastric cancer: a meta-analysis. *Gastroenterology* **145**(1):113–20.

Zhao Z, Yin Z, Zhao Q. (2017) Red and processed meat consumption and gastric cancer risk: a systematic review and meta-analysis. *Oncotarget* **8**(18):30563–75.

Zhou Y, Zhuang W, Hu W, Liu GJ, Wu TX, Wu XT. (2011) Consumption of large amounts of allium vegetables reduces risk of gastric cancer in a meta-analysis. *Gastroenterology* **141**(1):80–9.

Zhu H, Yang X, Zhang C, Zhu C, Tao G, Zhao L, Tang S, Shu Z, Cai J, Dai S, Qin Q, Xu L, Cheng H, Sun X. (2013) Red and processed meat intake is associated with higher gastric cancer risk: a meta-analysis of epidemiological observational studies. *PLoS One* **8**(8):e70955.

Stroke

Alexander DD, Miller PE, Vargas AJ, Weed DL, Cohen SS. (2016) Meta-analysis of egg consumption and risk of coronary heart disease and stroke. *J Am Coll Nutr* **35**(8):704–16.

De Goede J, Soedamah-Muthu SS, Pan A, Gijsbers L, Geleijnse JM. (2016) Dairy consumption and risk of stroke: a systematic review and updated dose-response meta-analysis of prospective cohort studies. *J Am Heart Assoc* **5**(5):pii: e002787.

Chen GC, Lv DB, Pang Z, Dong JY, Liu QF. (2013) Dietary fiber intake and stroke risk: a meta-analysis of prospective cohort studies. *Eur J Clin Nutr* **67**(1):96–100.

Chen GC, Lv DB, Pang Z, Liu QF. (2013) Red and processed meat consumption and risk of stroke: a meta-analysis of prospective cohort studies. *Eur J Clin Nutr* **67**(1):91–5.

Chen J, Huang Q, Shi W, Yang L, Chen J, Lan Q. (2016) Meta-analysis of the association between whole and refined grain consumption and stroke risk based on prospective cohort studies. *Asia Pac J Public Health* **28**(7):563–75.

Dauchet L, Amouyel P, Dallongeville J. (2005) Fruit and vegetable consumption and risk of stroke: a meta-analysis of cohort studies. *Neurology* **65**(8):1193–7.

Fang L, Li W, Zhang W, Wang Y, Fu S. (2015) Association between whole grain intake and stroke risk: evidence from a meta-analysis. *Int J Clin Exp Med* **8**(9):16978–83.

He FJ, Nowson Ca, MacGregor GA. (2016) Fruit and vegetable consumption and stroke: meta-analysis of cohort studies. *Lancet* **367**(9507):320–6.

Hu D, Huang J, Wang Y, Zhang D, Qu Y. (2014) Dairy foods and risk of stroke: a meta-analysis of prospective cohort studies. *Nutr Metab Cardiovasc Dis* **24**(5):460–9.

Hu D, Huang J, Wang Y, Zhang D, Qu Y. (2014) Fruits and vegetables consumption and risk of stroke: a meta-analysis of prospective cohort studies. *Stroke* **45**(6):1613–9.

Kaluza J, Wolk A, Larsson SC. (2012) Red meat consumption and risk of stroke: a meta-analysis of prospective studies. *Stroke* **43**(10):2556–60.

Larsson SC, Orsini N. (2011) Fish consumption and the risk of stroke: a dose-response meta-analysis. *Stroke* **42**(12):3621–3.

Li XY, Cai XL, Bian PD, Hu LR. (2012) High salt intake and stroke: meta-analysis of the epidemiologic evidence. *CNS Neurosci Ther* **18**(8):691–701.

Lou D, Li Y, Yan G, Bu J, Wang H. (2016) Soy consumption with risk of coronary heart disease and stroke: a meta-analysis of observational studies. *Neuroepidemiology* **46**(4):242–52.

Martinez-Gonzalez MA, Dominguez LJ, Delgado-Rodriguez M. (2014) Olive oil consumption and risk of CHD and/or stroke: a meta-analysis of case-control, cohort and intervention studies. *Br J Nutr* **112**(2):248–59.

Schwingshackl L, Hoffmann G. (2014) Monounsaturated fatty acids, olive oil and health status: a systematic review and meta-analysis of cohort studies. *Lipids Health Dis* **13**:154.

Shao C, Tang H, Zhao W, He J. (2016) Nut intake and stroke risk: a dose-response meta-analysis of prospective cohort studies. *Sci Rep* **6**:30394.

Shi ZQ, Tang JJ, Wu H, Xie CY, He ZZ. (2014) Consumption of nuts and legumes and risk of stroke: a meta-analysis of prospective studies. *Nutr Metab Cardiovasc Dis* **24**(12):1262–71.

Threapleton DE, Greenwood DC, Evans CE, Cleghorn CL, Nykjaer C, Woodhead C, Cade JE, Gale CP, Burley VJ. (2013) Dietary fiber intake and risk of first stroke: a systematic review and meta-analysis. *Stroke* **44**(5):1360–8.

Xun P, Qin B, Song Y, Nakamura Y, Kurth T, Yaemsiri S, Djousse L, He K. (2012) Fish consumption and risk of stroke and its subtypes: accumulative evidence from a meta-analysis of prospective cohort studies. *Eur J Clin Nutr* **66**(11):1199–207.

Yang C, Pan L, Sun C, Xi Y, Wang L, Li D. (2016) Red meat consumption and the risk of stroke: a dose-response meta-analysis of prospective cohort studies. *J Stroke Cerebrovasc Dis* 25(5):1177–86.

Zhao W, Tang H, Yang X, Luo X, Wang X, Shao C, He J. (2019) Fish consumption and stroke risk: a meta-analysis of prospective cohort studies. *J Stroke Cerebrovasc Dis* 28(3):604–11.

Zhang Y, Liu W, Liu D, Zhao T, Tian H. (2016) Efficacy of Aloe Vera supplementation on prediabetes and early non-treated diabetic patients: a systematic review and meta-analysis of randomized controlled trials. *Nutrients* 8(7):E388.

Zhang Z, Xu G, Wei Y, Zhu W, Liu X. (2105) Nut consumption and risk of stroke. *Eur J Epidemiol* 30(3):189–96.

Type 2 diabetes

Afshin A, Micha R, Khatibzadeh S, Mozaffarian D. (2104) Consumption of nuts and legumes and risk of incident ischemic heart disease, stroke, and diabetes: a systematic review and meta-analysis. *Am J Clin Nutr* 100(1):278–88.

Akilen R, Tsiami A, Devendra D, Robinson N. (2012) Cinnamon in glycaemic control: systematic review and meta analysis. *Clin Nutr* 31(5):609–15.

Allen RW, Schwartzman E, Baker WL, Coleman CI, Phung OJ. (2013) Cinnamon use in type 2 diabetes: an updated systematic review and meta-analysis. *Ann Fam Med* 11(5):452–9.

Alvarez-Bueno C, Cavero-Redondo I, Martinez-Vizcaino V, Sotos-Prieto M, Ruiz JR, Gil A. (2019) Effects of milk and dairy product consumption on type 2 diabetes: overview of systematic review an meta-analyses. *Adv Nutr* 10(suppl2):S154–S163.

Aune D, Keum N, Giovannucci E, Fadness LT, Boffetta P, Greenwood DC, Tonstad S, Vatten LJ, Riboli E, Norat T. (2016) Whole grain consumption and risk of cardiovascular disease, cancer, and all cause and cause specific mortality: systematic review and dose-response meta-analysis of prospective studies. *BMJ* 353:i2716.

Aune D, Norat T, Romundstad P, Vatten LJ. (2013) Dairy products and the risk of type 2 diabetes: a systematic review and dose-response meta-analysis of cohort studies. *Am J Clin Nutr* 98(4):1066–83.

Aune D, Norat T, Romundstad P, Vatten LJ. (2013) Whole grain and refined grain consumption and the risk of type 2 diabetes: a systematic review and dose-response meta-analysis of cohort studies. *Eur J Epidemiol* **28**(11):845–58.

Chanson-Rolle A, Meynier A, Aubin F, Lappi J, Poutanen K, Vinoy S, Braesco V. (2015) Systematic review and meta-analysis of human studies to support a quantitative recommendation for whole grain intake in relation to type 2 diabetes. *PLoS One* **10**(6):e0131377.

Carter P, Gray LJ, Troughton J, Khunti K, Davies MJ. (2010) Fruit and vegetable intake and incidence of type 2 diabetes mellitus: systematic review and meta-analysis. *BMJ* **341**:c4229.

Cooper AJ, Forouhi NG, Ye Z, Buijsse B, Arriola L, Balkau B, Barricarte A, Beulens JW, Boeing H, Buchner FL, Dahm CC, de Lauzon-Guillain B, Fagherazzi G, Franks PW, Gonzalez C, Grioni S, Kaaks R, Key TJ, Masala G, Navarro C, Nilsson P, Overvad K, Panico S, Ramon Quiros J, Rolandsson O, Roswall N, Sacerdote C, Sanchez MJ, Slimani N, Sluijs I, Spijkerman AM, Teucher B, Tjonneland A, Tumino R, Sharp SJ, Langenberg C, Feskens EJ, Riboli E, Wareham NJ. (2012) InterAct Consortium. Fruit and vegetable intake and type 2 diabetes: EPIC-InterAct prospective study and meta-analysis. *Eur J Nutr* **66**(10):1082–92.

Davis PA, Yokoyama W. (2011) Cinnamon intake lowers fasting blood glucose: meta-analysis. *J Med Food* **14**(9):884–9.

Dick WR, Fletcher EA, Shah SA. (2016) Reduction of fasting blood glucose and hemoglobin A1c using oral aloe vera: a meta-analysis. *J Altern Complement Med* **22**(6):450–7.

Djousse L, Khawaja OA, Gaziano JM. (2016) Egg consumption and risk of type 2 diabetes: a meta-analysis of prospective studies. *Am J Clin Nutr* **103**(2):474–80.

Esponsito K, Kastorini CM, Panagiotakos DB, Giugliano D. (2010) Prevention of type 2 diabetes by dietary patterns: a systematic review of prospective studies and meta-analysis. *Metab Syndr Relat Disord* **8**(6):471–6.

Fretts AM, Follis JL, Nettleton JA, Lemaitre RN, Ngwa JS, Wojczynski MK, Kalafati IP, Varga TV, Frazier-Wood AC, Houston DK, Lahti J, Ericson U, van den Hooven EH, Mikkila V, Kiefte-de Jong JC,

Mozaffarian D, Rice K, Renstrom F, North KE, McKeown NM, Feitosa MF, Kanoni S, Smith CE, Garcia ME, Tiainen AM, Sonestedt E, Manichaikul A, van Rooij FJ, Dimitriou M, Raitakari O, Pankow JS, Djousse L, Province MA, Hu FB, Lai CQ, Keller MF, Perala MM, Rotter JI, Hofman A, Graff M, Kohonen M, Mukamal K, Johansson I, Ordovas JM, Liu Y, Mannisto S, Uitterlinden AG, Deloukas P, Seppala I, Psaty BM, Cupples LA, Borecki IB, Franks PW, Arnett DK, Nalls MA, Eriksson JG, Ortho-Melander M, Franco OH, Lehtimaki T, Dedoussis GV, Meigs JB, Siscovick DS. (2015) Consumption of meat is associated with higher fasting glucose and insulin concentrations regardless of glucose and insulin genetic risk scores: the meta-analysis of 50,345 Caucasians. *Am J Clin Nutr* **102**(5):1266–78.

Gijsbers L, Ding EL, Malik VS, de Goede J, Geleijnse JM, Soedamah-Muthu SS. (2016) Consumption of dairy foods and diabetes incidence: a dose-response meta-analysis of observational studies. *Am J Clin Nutr* **103**(4):1111–24.

Greenwood DC, Threapleton DE, Evans CE, Cleghorn CL, Nykjaer C, Woodhead C, Burley VJ. (2014) Association between sugar-sweetened and artificially sweetened soft drinks and type 2 diabetes: systematic review and dose-response meta-analysis of prospective studies. *Br J Nutr* **112**(5):725–34.

Guo K, Zhou Z, Jiang Y, Li W, Li Y. (2015) Meta-analysis of prospective studies on the effects of nut consumption on hypertension and type 2 diabetes mellitus. *J Diabetes* **7**(2):202–12.

Guo X, Yang B, Tan J, Jiang J, Li D. (2016) Associations of dietary intakes of anthocyanins and berry fruits with risk of type 2 diabetes mellitus: a systematic review and meta-analysis of prospective cohort studies. *Eur J Clin Nutr* **70**(12):1360–67.

Guo XF, Yang B, Tang J, Jiang JJ, Li D. (2017) Apple and pear consumption and type 2 diabetes mellitus: a meta-analysis of prospective cohort studies. *Food Funct* **8**(3):927–34.

Hausenblas HA, Schoulda JA, Smoliga JM. (2015) Resveratol treatment as an adjunct to pharmacological management in type 2 diabetes mellitus — systematic review and meta-analysis. *Mol Nutr Food Res* **59**(1):147–59.

He LX, Zhao J, Huang YS, Li Y. (2016) The difference between oats and beta-glucan extract intake in the management of HbA1c, fasting glucose and insulin sensitivity: a meta-analysis of randomized controlled trials. *Food Funct* 7(3):1413–28.

Hou LQ, Liu YH, Zhang YY. (2015) Garlic intake lowers fasting blood glucose: meta-analysis of randomized controlled trials. *Asia Pac J Clin Nutr* 24(4):575–82.

Hou Q, Li Y, Li L, Cheng G, Sun X, Li S, Tian H. (2015) The metabolic effects of oats intake in patients with type 2 diabetes: a systematic review and meta-analysis. *Nutrients* 7(12):10369–87.

Hu EA, Pan A, Malik V, Sun Q. (2012) White rice consumption and risk of type 2 diabetes: meta-analysis and systematic review. *BMJ* 344:e1454.

Hu YM, Zhou F, Yuan Y, Xu YC. (2017) Effects of probiotics supplement in patients with type 2 diabetes mellitus: a meta-analysis of randomized trials. *Med Clin (Barc)* 148(8):362–70.

Imamura F, O'Connor L, Ye Z, Mursu J, Hayashino Y, Bhupathiraju SN, Forouhi NG. (2015) Consumption of sugar sweetened beverages, artificially sweetened beverages, and fruit juice and incidence of type 2 diabetes: systematic review, meta-analysis, and estimation of population attributable fraction. *BMJ* 351:h3576.

Imamura F, O'Connor L, Ye Z, Mursu J, Hayashino Y, Bhupathiraju SN, Forouhi NG. (2016) Consumption of sugar sweetened beverages, artificially sweetened beverages, and fruit juice and incidence of type 2 diabetes: systematic review, meta-analysis, and estimation of population attributable fraction. *Br J Sports Med* 50(8):496–504.

InterAct Consortium. (2015) Dietary fibre and incidence of type 2 diabetes in eight European countries: the EPIC-InterAct Study and the meta-analysis of prospective studies. *Diabetologia* 58(7):1394–408.

Jannasch F, Kroger J, Schulze MB. (2017) Dietary patterns and type 2 diabetes: a systematic literature review and meta-analysis of prospective studies. *J Nutr* 147(6):1174–82.

Jia X, Zhong L, Song Y, Hu Y, Wang G, Sun S. (2016) Consumption of citrus and cruciferous vegetables with incident type 2 diabetes mellitus based on a meta-analysis of prospective study. *Prim Care Diabetes* 10(4):272–80.

Knott C, Bell S, Britton A. (2015) Alcohol consumption and the risk of type 2 diabetes: a systematic review and dose-response meta-analysis of more than 1.9 million individuals from 38 observational studies. *Diabetes Care* **38**(9):1804–12.

Li C, Li X, Han H, Cui H, Peng M, Wang G, Wang Z. (2016) Effect of probiotics on metabolic profiles in type 2 diabetes mellitus: a meta-analysis of randomized, controlled trials. *Medicine (Baltimore)* **95**(26):e4088.

Li M, Fan Y, Zhang X, Hou W, Tang Z. (2014) Fruit and vegetable intake and risk of type 2 diabetes mellitus: meta-analysis of prospective cohort studies. *BMJ Open* **4**(11):e005497.

Li S, Miao S, Huang Y, Liu Z, Tian H, Yin X, Tang W, Steffen LM, Xi B. (2015) Fruit intake decreases risk of incident type 2 diabetes: an updated meta-analysis. *Endocrine* **48**(2):454–60.

Li W, Ruan W, Peng Y, Wang D. (2018) Soy and the risk of type 2 diabetes mellitus: a systematic review and meta-analysis of observational studies. *Diabetes Res Clin Pract* **137**:190–9.

Li Y, Wang C, Huai Q, Guo F, Liu L, Feng R, Sun C. (2016) Effects of tea or tea extract on metabolic profiles in patients with type 2 diabetes mellitus: a meta-analysis of ten randomized controlled trials. *Diabetes Meta Res Rev* **32**(1):2–10.

Li Y, Zhou C, Zhou X, Li L. (2013) Egg consumption and risk of cardiovascular diseases and diabetes: a meta-analysis. *Atherosclerosis* **229**(2):524–30.

Liu K, Zhou R, Wang B, Mi MT. (2014) Effect of resveratrol on glucose control and insulin sensitivity: a meta-analysis of 11 randomized controlled trials. *Am J Clin Nutr* **99**(6):1510–9.

Liu Y, Li J, Wang T, Wang Y, Zhao L, Fang Y. (2107) The effect of genistein on glucose control and insulin sensitivity in postmenopausal women: a meta-analysis. *Maturitas* **97**:44–52.

Luo C, Zhang Y, Ding Y, Shan Z, Chen S, Yu M, Hu FB, Liu L. (2014) Nut consumption and risk of type 2 diabetes, cardiovascular disease, and all-cause mortality: a systematic review and meta-analysis. *Am J Clin Nutr* **100**(1):256–69.

Malik VS, Popkin BM, Bray GA, Despres JP, Willett WC, Hu FB. (2010) Sugar-sweetened beverages and risk of metabolic syndrome and type 2 diabetes: a meta-analysis. *Diabetes Care* **33**(11):2477–83.

McRae MP. (2017) Health benefits of dietary whole grains: an umbrella review of meta-analyses. *J Chiropr Med* **16**(1):10–8.

Micha R, Wallace SK, Mozaffarian D. (2010) Red and processed meat consumption and risk of incident coronary heart disease, stroke, and diabetes mellitus: a systematic review and meta-analysis. *Circulation* 121(21):2271–83.

Mohammadi-Sartang M, Sohrabi Z, Barati-Boldaji R, Raeisi-Dehkordi H, Mazloom Z. (2018) Flaxseed supplementation on glucose control and insulin sensitivity: a systematic review and meta-analysis of 25 randomized, placebo-controlled trials. *Nutr Rev* 76(2):125–39.

Nettleton JA, McKeown NM, Kanoni S, Lemaitre RN, Hivert MF, Ngwa J, van Rooij FJ, Sonestedt E, Wojczynski MK, Ye Z, Tanaka T, Garcia M, Anderson JS, Follis JL, Djousse L, Mukamal K, Papoutsakis C, Mozaffarian D, Zillikens MC, Bandinelli S, Bennett AJ, Borecki IB, Feitosa MF, Ferrucci L, Forouhi NG, Groves CJ, Hallmans G, Harris T, Hofman A, Houston DK, Hu FB, Johansson I, Kritchevsky SB, Langenberg C, Launer L, Liu Y, Loos RJ, Nalls M, Orho-Melander M, Renstrom F, Rice K, Riserus U, Rolandsson O, Rotter JI, Saylor G, Sijbrands EJ, Sjogren P, Smith A, Steingrimsdottir L, Uitterlinden AG, Wareham NJ, Prokopenko I, Pankow JS, van Duijn CM, Florez JC, Witteman JC, MAGIC investigators, Dupuis J, Dedoussis GV, Ordovas JM, Ingelsson E, Cupples L, Siscovick DS, Franks PW, Meigs JB. (2010) Interactions of dietary whole-grain intake with fasting glucose- and insulin-related genetic loci in individuals of European descent: the meta-analysis of 14 cohort studies. *Diabetes Care* 33(12): 2684–91.

Neuenschwander M, Ballon A, Weber KS, Norat T, Aune D, Schwingshackl L, Schlesinger S. (2019) Role of diet in type 2 diabetes incidence: umbrella review of meta-analyses of observational studies. *BMJ* 366:l2368.

Pan A, Sun Q, Bernstein AM, Schulze MB, Manson JE, Willett WC, Hu FB. (2011) Red meat consumption and risk of type 2 diabetes: 3 cohorts of US adults and an updated meta-analysis, *Am J Clin Nutr* 94(4):1088–96.

Post RE, Mainous AG 3rd, King DE, Simpson KN. (2012) Dietary fiber for the treatment of type 2 diabetes mellitus: a meta-analysis. *J Am Board Fam Med* 25(1):16–23.

Qian F, Korat AA, Malik V, Hu FB. (2016) Metabolic effects of mono-unsaturated fatty acid-enriched diets compared with carbohydrate or polyunsaturated fatty acid-enriched diets in patients with type 2 diabetes: a systematic review and meta-analysis of randomized controlled trials. *Diabetes Care* **39**(8):1448–57.

Rehackova L, Arnott B, Araujo-Soares V, Adamson AA, Taylor R, Sniehotta FF. (2016) Efficacy and acceptability of very low energy diets in overweight and obese people with type 2 diabetes mellitus: a systematic review with meta-analyses. *Diabet Med* **33**(5):580–91.

Ruan Y, Sun J, He J, Chen F, Chen R, Chen H. (2015) Effect of probiotics on glycemic control: a systematic review and meta-analysis of randomized, controlled trials. *PLoS One* **10**(7):e0132121.

Samah S, Ramasamy K, Lim SM, Neoh CF. (2016) Probiotics for the management of type 2 diabetes mellitus: a systematic review and meta-analysis. *Diabetes Res Clin Pract* **118**:172–82.

Schwingshackl L, Hoffmann G, Lampousi AM, Knuppel S, Igbal K, Schwedhelm C, Bechthold A, Schlesinger S, Boeing H. (2017) Food groups and risk of type 2 diabetes mellitus: a systematic review and meta-analysis of prospective studies. *Eur J Epidemiol* **32**(5):363–75.

Schwingshackl L, Lampousi AM, Portillo MP, Romaguera D, Hoffmann G, Boeing H. (2017) Olive oil in the prevention and management of type 2 diabetes mellitus: a systematic review and meta-analysis of cohort studies and intervention trials. *Nutr Diabetes* **7**(4):e262.

Silva FM, Kramer CK, de Almeida JC, Steemburgo T, Gross JL, Azevedo MJ. (2013) Fiber intake and glycemic control in patients with type 2 diabetes mellitus: a systematic review with meta-analysis of randomized controlled trials. *Nutr Rev* **71**(12):790–801.

Snorgaard O, Poulsen GM, Andersen HK, Astrup A. (2017) Systematic review and meta-analysis of dietary carbohydrate restriction in patients with type 2 diabetes. *BMJ Open Diabetes Res Care* **5**(1):e000354.

Suksomboon N, Poolsup N, Punthanitisarn S. (2016) Effect of aloe vera on glycaemic control in prediabetes and type 2 diabetes: a systematic review and meta-analysis. *J Clin Pharm Ther* **41**(2):180–8.

Sun J, Buys NJ. (2016) Glucose- and glycaemic factor-lowering effects of probiotics on diabetes: a meta-analysis of randomized placebo-controlled trials. *Br J Nutr* **115**(7):1167–77.

Tamez M, Virtanen JK, Lajous M. (2016) Egg consumption and risk of incident type 2 diabetes: a dose-response meta-analysis of prospective cohort studies. *Br J Nutr* **115**(12):2212–8.

Tong X, Dong JY, Wu ZW, Li W, Qin LQ. (2011) Dairy consumption and risk of type 2 diabetes mellitus: a meta-analysis of cohort studies. *Eur J Clin Nutr* 65(9):1027–31.

Viana LV, Gross JL, Azevedo MJ. (2014) Dietary intervention in patients with gestational diabetes mellitus: a systematic review and meta-analysis of randomized clinical trials on maternal and newborn outcomes. *Diabetes Care* 37(12):3345–55.

Viguiliouk E, Kendall CW, Blanco Mejia S, Cozma AI, Ha V, Mirrahimi A, Jayalath VH, Augustin LS, Chiavaroli L, Leiter LA, de Souza RJ, Jenkins DJ, Sievenpiper JL. (2014) Effect of tree nuts on glycemic control in diabetes: a systematic review and meta-analysis of randomized controlled dietary trials. *PLoS One* 9(7):e103376.

Wallin A, Forouhi NG, Wolk A, Larsson SC. (2016) Egg consumption and risk of type 2 diabetes: a prospective study and dose-response meta-analysis. *Diabetologia* 59(6):1204–13.

Wanders AJ, Boom WAM, Zock PL, Geleijnse JM, Brouwer IA, Alssema M. (2019) Plant-based polyunsaturated fatty acids and markers of glucose metabolism and insulin resistance: a meta-analysis of randomized controlled feeding trials. *BMJ Open Diabetes Res Care* 7(1):e000585.

Wang M, Yu M, Fang L, Hu RY. (2015) Association between sugar-sweetened beverages and type 2 diabetes: a meta-analysis. *J Diabetes Investig* 6(3):360–6.

Wang PY, Fang JC, Gao ZH, Zhang C, Xie SY. (2016) Higher intake of fruits, vegetables or their fiber reduces the risk of type 2 diabetes: the meta-analysis. *J Diabetes Investig* 7(1):56–69.

Wu L, Wang Z, Zhu J, Murad AL, Prokop LJ, Murad MH. (2015) Nut consumption and risk of cancer and type 2 diabetes: a systematic review and meta-analysis. *Nutr Rev* 73(7):409–25.

Wu Y, Zhang D, Jiang X, Jiang W. (2015) Fruit and vegetable consumption and risk of type 2 diabetes mellitus: a dose-response meta-analysis of prospective cohort studies. *Nutr Metab Cardiovasc Dis* 25(2):140–7.

Xi B, Li S, Liu Z, Tian H, Yin X, Huai P, Tang W, Zhou D, Steffen LM. (2014) Intake of fruit juice and incidence of type 2 diabetes: a systematic review and meta-analysis. *PLoS One* 9(3):e93471.

Yakoob MY, Shi P, Willett WC, Rexrode KM, Campos H, Orav EJ, Ju FB, Mozaffarian D. (2016) Circulating biomarkers of dairy fat and risk of incident diabetes mellitus among men and women in the United States in two large prospective cohorts. *Circulation* **133**(17):1645–54.

Ye EQ, Chacko SA, Chou EL, Kugizaki M, Liu S. (2012) Greater whole-grain intake is associated with lower risk of type 2 diabetes, cardiovascular disease and weight gain. *J Nutr* **142**(7):1304–13.

Yokoyama Y, Barnard ND, Levin SM, Watanabe M. (2014) Vegetarian diets and glycemic control in diabetes: a systematic review and meta-analysis. *Cardiovasc Diagn Ther* **4**(5):373–82.

Zhang Y, Liu W, Liu D, Zhao T, Tian H. (2016) Efficacy of Aloe Vera supplementation on prediabetes and early non-treated diabetic patients: a systematic review and meta-analysis of randomized controlled trials. *Nutrients* **8**(7):E388

Zhou D, Yu H, He F, Reilly KH, Zhang J, Li S, Zhang T, Wang B, Ding Y, Xi B. (2014) Nut consumption in relation to cardiovascular disease risk and type 2 diabetes: a systematic review and meta-analysis of prospective studies. *Am J Clin Nutr* **100**(1):270–7.

Index

Made in the USA
Middletown, DE
21 March 2023